Mad by the Millions

To Prof. Sturdy.

Thank you for all the support and inspiration.

Harry AUG. 2023

Culture and Psychiatry

Edited by Neil Aggarwal

'Aṣfūriyyeh: A History of Madness, Modernity, and War in the Middle East by Joelle M. Abi-Rached

Mad by the Millions: Mental Disorders and the Early Years of the World Health Organization by Harry Yi-Jui Wu

Mad by the Millions

Mental Disorders and the Early Years of the World Health Organization

Harry Yi-Jui Wu

The MIT Press
Cambridge, Massachusetts
London, England

This book was set in Stone Serif and Stone Sans by Westchester Publishing Services. Printed and bound in the United States of America.

Library of Congress Cataloging-in-Publication Data

Names: Wu, Harry Yi-Jui, 1978- author.
Title: Mad by the millions : mental disorders and the early years of the World Health Organization / Harry Yi-Jui Wu.
Description: Cambridge, Massachusetts : The MIT Press, [2021] | Series: Culture and psychiatry | Includes bibliographical references and index.
Identifiers: LCCN 2020020601 | ISBN 9780262045384 (paperback)
Subjects: LCSH: World Health Organization. | Mental health--International cooperation. | Mental illness--Measurement. | Social psychiatry. | World health.
Classification: LCC RA790.5 .W8 2021 | DDC 362.1--dc23
LC record available at https://lccn.loc.gov/2020020601

10 9 8 7 6 5 4 3 2 1

Contents

1964
- Ten-Year Plan in Psychiatric initiated
- Asylums
- John and Lorna Wing conducted Camberwell study
- Tsung-yi Lin became Medical Officer in the WHO's Mental Health Section

1966
- Cultural Revolution began in China (1966)
- IPSS (1966-1973)

1969
- Tsung-yi Lin left WHO
- B. Lebedev became chief of MHU (1969-70)

1971
- Taiwan left WHO
- F. Hassler became chief of MHU (1971-74)

1972
- People's Republic of China joined WHO

1974
- Norman Sartorius became chief of Office of Mental Health (1974-77)

1976
- Cultural Revolution ended in China

1977
- Norman Sartorius became Director of Division of Mental Health (1977-94)
- Kleinman proposed New Cross-cultural Psychiatry (1977)A. Kleinman proposed New Cross-cultural Psychiatry

1978
- DOSMED study (1978-1980)

1979
- ICD-9
- First CCMD published in China
- The International Conference on Primary Health Care, Alma-Ata Declaration of WHO

1990
- ICD-10

1991
- Sickness and Healing: An Anthropological Perspective (Kleinman, 1991)
- USSR ended

1994
- J. A. Costa e Silva became Director of Division of Mental Health (1994-98)

1996
- ICD-8a

1999
- B. Saraceno became Director of the Department of Mental Health

2007
- The Lancet published Global Mental Health series

2013
- DSM-5

2018
- ICD-11

were also employed to help insurance companies reap profits. Universal standards were thus based on a unity of purpose rather than on scientific investigation.

The universality of mental disorders has similarly been long debated. The debate can be best understood by the conflict between two main classification systems: those codified in the *Diagnostic and Statistical Manual of Mental Disorders* and in the *International Classification of Diseases*.[2] In this book, though, the focus is broader than the question of commonality across human populations. Disagreements over the loosening of the diagnostic criteria that apply to mental disorders have challenged a classification that some critics consider responsible for expanding the global pharmaceutical industry.[3] In May 2013, for example, two weeks before the release of the cutting-edge fifth edition of the *Diagnostic and Statistical Manual of Mental Disorders* (*DSM-5*), the National Institute of Mental Health (NIMH), the world's largest funding agency for research into mental health, withdrew its support for the manual. The director of NIMH, Thomas R. Insel, emphasized that the Institute would no longer fund research projects that relied on the new *DSM* criteria. Instead, he proposed to move away from the *DSM* system and adopt another framework, the NIMH's own Research Domain Criteria, RDoC, to explore different dimensions of mental disorders. NIMH was not alone in its criticisms of *DSM-5*.[4] In his best-selling book *Saving Normal*, Allen Frances, chair of *DSM-5*'s predecessor, *DSM-IV*, and professor emeritus of psychiatry at Duke University, condemned the new *DSM*, stating that its task force fell short in collecting substantial evidence to support its profiles of mental disorders and their classification.[5] He further criticized the new approach for benefiting pharmaceutical companies, allowing them the liberty to treat a wide spectrum of mental disorders without constraints and resulting in unlimited use of medication for a much wider range of conditions.

The response to *DSM*'s alternative—different revisions of chapter V of the *International Classification of Diseases* (*ICD*)—has been more benign. It did not receive much criticism as it is less involved with pharmaceutical industries. However, debates on *ICD* categories also have a long history. The *ICD* existed long before the World Health Organization (WHO) was formed. Its earlier incarnation, the *International List of Causes of Death*, first emerged in 1893 for the convenience of international trade. This ever longer list of diseases was compiled to monitor the spread of predominantly infectious diseases through the circulation of commodities and the movement of travelers.

In 1946, the WHO took over the painstaking work of classifying causes of death. The list further included what causes diseases. Now written by the WHO, the modern *ICD* established a standardized system, including a glossary and methods to measure mental disorders that are "internationally acceptable and capable of uniform application."[6] While clinicians and scientists in various nations were working to establish a complete list of diseases, the Interim Commission of the WHO included mental disorders in the discussion at its June-July 1946 International Health Conference in New York City. Mental disorders then appeared for the first time in the sixth revision of the *ICD*. That list, however, was short and simple, consisting of only a handful of disorders related to psychosis, neurosis, and mental deficiency.[7] Not until the late 1950s, when the Mental Health Unit of the WHO sought to produce demographic data and an all-encompassing system for measuring mental disorders, did the *ICD* develop a diagnostic instrument for worldwide use.

From 1946 to 2018, from *ICD-6* to *ICD-11*, the number of mental disorders in both *DSM* and *ICD* classification systems increased rapidly. The increase can be attributed to the discovery of new disease types, subtler descriptions of their presentations, and greater attention to their causations. As the Maudsley-trained Bulgarian psychiatrist Assen Jablensky, who chaired the development of the *ICD-11* diagnostic criteria for mental disorders, noted in 2016, much of the progress toward understanding psychiatric disorders had until then been achieved by "splitting rather than by lumping."[8] This process contradicts the WHO's original attempt to produce a simple diagnostic system. Users of *ICD-10* had also disparaged its scientific value and global applicability, and further calls had been made to improve the classification system in *ICD-11*, to provide clinicians and researchers better information about causation, clinical presentation, and treatment options for mental disorders. In June 2018, *ICD-11* was published with updated scientific content and less complex information. Clinicians and scientists of UN member states found it useful to prepare for implementation, including translating the system into their own languages. They hoped that the eleventh revision would be in use at the beginning of 2022.

In the 1990s, calls had multiplied to reform mental health at the global level and to "decolonize" the universal approach to mental disorders. Alongside attempts to adapt "non-Western" metrics for mental disorders, the push to reform mental health was part of the evolution of psychiatric classification. "New cross-cultural psychiatry" sought a culturally sensitive approach that looked at contextual influences on the ways mental disorders were experienced, explained, and managed.[9] The WHO's Mental Health Gap Action Program aimed to scale up mental health services in low- and middle-income countries. By stressing scientific evidence and human rights, the movement for global mental health attempted, through volunteerism and cross-disciplinary collaboration, to improve services that were still scarce in underdeveloped regions.[10] From the immediate postwar period to the millennium, these approaches gradually became more and more "bottom up," emphasizing the needs of people affected by mental symptoms, especially those in poorly resourced areas. They also became more "democratic," drawing on the perspectives of different scientific groups and professionals. These campaigns pointed out not only the inadequacy of existing resources for people living with mental health problems and for psychosocially disabled individuals and populations, but also the inadequacy of existing tools for understanding mental disorders worldwide. Beyond disputes over *DSM* or *ICD*, they indicated as well the consideration and development of interventions beyond diagnosis.

I studied medicine in Taiwan, an island with a health system that includes public and private services at all levels. Toward the end of the nineteenth century, different colonizers still deemed it unsuitable for dwelling because of its hot weather and diseased condition. Now, it has its own complete associated regulations for health and medical education. Its National Health Insurance scheme has been praised as the top model in Asia, and it attracts health authorities from various countries.[11] Despite losing its seat at the WHO in 1971, Taiwan continued to adopt and implement the best knowledge technologies in a social context where the scientific and medical community is modern and considers itself Westernized.[12] Halfway through my specialty training in psychiatry, I pursued further study in England, in the history of medicine. I came to understand that modern psychiatry and many medical specialties in Taiwan differed in their early development from the development of these disciplines in other countries in the Asia-Pacific region. Taiwan developed a nationwide health infrastructure and implemented a training system based on national board certification committees. In the past half century, modern medicine in Taiwan has progressed rapidly. The medical profession takes part in international medical research activities and international medical conferences, and offers high-quality health services for allied countries, all without being granted a seat at the WHO. When I took part in these conferences, I found myself undeterred from articulating the language and knowledge discussed on those occasions because Taiwan's comprehensive medical education system and its advanced treatment and care systems have made its doctors no different from those in the Western world.

In the training program for my psychiatry residency, one of the most important competencies for the final certification examination was the ability to formulate a proper diagnosis for a real patient according to *DSM* criteria. These criteria are all available in Chinese. In the transition from *DSM-IV* to *DSM-5*, practitioners feared controversies over standards. Yet, surprisingly, the shift went peacefully, and *DSM-5* presented few problems in coding conditions for health insurance in Taiwan. However, the adoption of the *ICD* codes did not happen so quietly in many countries. The slow adoption of the *ICD* codes reflects two major problems that countries face in the big picture of global health. First, social, economic, and cultural conditions in various parts of the world are too different to apply a single standard. Second, the validity and reliability of the internationally ratified system for disease classification are still questionable. Health systems in most developing countries have made efforts to adopt the *ICD* codes. In some countries, however, cultural conditions spur debate over disease classification. Such dilemmas reflect earlier arguments about whether mental disorders are universal, or at least comparable in their incidence and prevalence. Early in 1920s, for example, C. G. Seligman (1873–1940), a physician-anthropologist, famously argued that severe mental illness was unknown in early-contact New Guinea, which he called a "stone-age population," except in places marked by Westernization.[13] His claim was soon disproved after other anthropologists found mental illness hidden in local patterns of ritual performance and manifested differently than in the West. Despite the consensus that all human beings can suffer from mental conditions of some form, debates over the universality or heterogeneity of mental disorders never stop.

Recognizing that people might experience similar mental disorders across cultures, scientists collated a robust international diagnostic system in the second half of the twentieth century. In China, however, there were calls for a specifically Chinese classification of mental disorders.[14] The claim to essential difference implies that the international system falls short in accounting for needs and conditions in some parts of the world. Although research in psychiatric sciences was suspended in China during the decade of the Cultural Revolution (1966–1976), psychiatrists managed to develop an infrastructure for mental health, including China's own diagnostic system, which was established during the reforms of the late 1970s to meet the needs of those lacking care. Three major changes have since appeared. In the early 1980s, after having ignored China for almost three decades, the WHO established a center in Beijing to promote its work and to analyze the compatibility of the Chinese system with the *ICD*. These efforts challenged the notion that science is neutral. Rather, they suggested the outcome and content of scientific inquiry were determined by structural conditions, political arrangements, and institutional concerns. Recently, China has planned to abandon its *Chinese Classification for Mental Disorders* (*CCMD*).[15] Obviously, employing the *ICD* system helps China better connect with international scientific and medical communities.

The comparability of mental conditions across different cultures is conveyed in the 1959 French new wave film *Hiroshima Mon Amour*, which illustrates the trauma produced by World War II:

He: You saw nothing in Hiroshima. Nothing.

She: I saw everything. Everything.

She: The hospital, for instance, I saw it. I'm sure I did. There is a hospital in Hiroshima. How could I help seeing it?

He: You did not see the hospital in Hiroshima. You saw nothing in Hiroshima.

...

She: I saw the patience, the innocence, the apparent meekness with which the temporary survivors of Hiroshima adapted themselves to a fate so unjust that the imagination, normally so fertile, cannot conceive it.

He: Nothing. You know nothing.[16]

Through this scene, the playwright and novelist Marguerite Duras and the director Alain Resnais explore the inscrutability of communication between psychological subjects. The movie begins with a scene of two bodies entangled with each other in the dark. The scene describes a romantic rendezvous between a Japanese architect (He) and a French actress (She) temporarily working in Hiroshima on a film about a peace mission. The encounter triggers memories about her affair with a German soldier in Nevers during

World War II—and a chain of events she had never told anyone else about. The soldier was killed on the day the city was liberated, and she suffered from public disgrace and imprisonment before she finally left for Paris when the war ended. The film asks a series of questions about the truth claims of memories and the representation of witnesses. It further questions whether individuals from different cultures can communicate their traumatic pasts to one another and achieve a full understanding. For example, the Japanese architect refuses to believe that the actress could empathize with the devastation he witnessed in Hiroshima. By the end of the film, the cultural clash between the architect and the actress is resolved through love.

Quite fascinatingly, the film raises a question related to the inquiries of psychiatric scientists at the time. Toward the end of the 1950s, mental health experts at the WHO were attempting to demonstrate the commonality, comparability, or in more professional terms, "commensurability" of psychiatric disorders worldwide. On a practical level, they were looking for a scientific method that would, if not prove, then at least inquire into the plausibility of such a concept. Their question coincided with Duras and Resnais's fictional sketch, but it took decades for them to find answers.

This book seeks, in part, to explain the history of the WHO's mental health classification system. Unlike most critiques of psychiatric classifications, I do not haggle over the oppressive nature of such systems. Rather, the book explains the immense global effort involved in the WHO's work on social psychiatry and subsequent efforts to classify diseases, and the writing of chapter V of *ICD-9* (1975), which emerged from debates ranging from the late 1940s to the early 1970s. Such efforts not only demonstrated the process by which mental disorders were "globalized," but also represented an epic project whose purpose was decolonization. Through the project, the WHO sought to improve the mental health of desolate war victims and to establish the infrastructure of psychiatry in countries where professionals, resources, and even working languages were absent.

The WHO's early definition of social psychiatry emerged roughly as deinstitutionalization began, primarily in the West, in the decades after World War II. This period saw a crucial transformation in the relationship between society and the mentally ill, as people questioned whether the mentally ill had to be secluded and whether secure institutions were the most therapeutically valuable spaces for recovery.[17] Taking a similar "inclusive approach," the WHO's definition of "social psychiatry" implied that everyone in the world could become mentally ill. The newfangled discipline referred to "the preventive and curative measures which are directed towards the fitting of the individual for a satisfactory and useful life in terms of his own social environment."[18] The definition includes a conceptual approach to mental disorders regarding the social determinants of "diseases," instruments for measurement, and a classification system as an end product. This definition further reflects the assumptions of a group of psychiatrists that mental disorders result from both inner conflicts and external influences, and that mental disorders are preventable. By the time the WHO implemented its social psychiatry project, the focus was twofold: first, to apply the techniques of epidemiology to study profiles of mental disorders; second, to treat mental disorders as actual diseases shaped by their own course, social determinants, and processes of causation.

The WHO's effort appeared almost half a century before the appeals of medical anthropologists during the 1980s and 1990s to study local biologies, the medical hermeneutics of bodies, and mental disorders in various cultures. Criticizing the use of universal criteria, the medical anthropologists instead accentuated the meanings of diseases, including the rational, irrational, and even moral dimension of interpretations among various individuals and communities.[19] But the WHO's bold and ambitious project to designate the universality of mental disorders coincided with the mushrooming identification of culture-bound syndromes in different worldwide surveys in the 1960s. The project also appeared as the discipline of transcultural psychiatry was taking shape and as mental disorders were becoming a global burden after the devastations of World War II. This period was marked by a global demand to study the common language of psychiatry, while psychiatrists worldwide were looking for robust evidence to support the application of scientific methods and principles in social psychiatry. In the post-World War II period, mental health came to be treated as a global public health issue through a newly established international health organization.

Once an Internationally Shared Vision

"Mad by the millions" is a direct translation of *folie à millions*, a phrase used by the eminent psychoanalyst and social critic Erich Fromm, in response to the need to understand mental disorders after World War II. In his 1941 book *Escape from Freedom*, Fromm explored the psychosocial conditions that developed alongside the rise of Nazism and other types of authoritarianism. In 1955, Fromm published *The Sane Society* as the sequel to *Escape from Freedom*. In it he critiqued the rise of capitalism as a threat to the human psyche, and he deciphered the immense anxiety human beings experience when they conform to modern society. In a way, he tried to answer the question Sigmund Freud raised in his *Civilization and Its Discontents*: "If the evolution of civilization has such a far-reaching similarity with the development of an individual, and if the same methods are employed in both, would not the diagnosis be justified that many systems of civilization—or epochs of it—possibly even the whole of humanity—have become 'neurotic' under the pressure of the civilizing trends?"[20]

Today, in contrast, the proliferating scholarly and popular accounts accuse the mental health enterprise of expanding its power to medicalize daily life.[21] Following Michel Foucault, much analysis over the past decade has focused on the power that psychiatry and its related industries hold over the human psyche and human behavior. For example, Robert Whitaker's *Anatomy of an Epidemic* criticizes psychiatry as an enterprise hijacked by capitalism. The medical journalist argues that mental illness has become much more prevalent in the United States since the biological revolution in psychiatry in the 1950s and that pharmaceutical industries are responsible.[22] Gary Greenberg's *The Book of Woe* disparages the *DSM* system, arguing that it may help people cope better with life but also leads to a reductionism that insults a sense of self.[23] Cultural historian Michael E. Staub, in *Madness Is Civilization*, finds psychiatrists in postwar America repressing rational reactions to crude social conditions, thus creating and exacerbating mental disorders. In Ethan Watters's *Crazy Like Us*, Watters sees global psychiatry being influenced by the United States through the dissemination of the *DSM*.[24] Recent criticism of global psychiatry includes Bruce Cohen's Marxist take on present-day psychiatric discourse. He argues that neoliberal capitalism, through the manipulations of big pharma, has extended psychiatry's hegemonic reach.[25] Employing postcolonial theories, China Mills introduces the terms "global psychiatrization" and "psychiatric colonization" to question the social and cultural justice underlying global psychiatry.[26]

These critiques, though emerging in different times, sketch a picture in which psychiatry is a hegemonic and inhumane science in service to state authorities or global big pharma. They, however, ignore that a "globalized psyche" was in high demand in the precarious postwar era. From the late

1940s to the early 1970s, psychiatrists, like many medical and social scientists, shared a vision of the universality of mental disorders that differed greatly from present-day critiques of the globalization of mental illness and the role of big pharma. Instead, they tried to understand these conditions on the basis of a lack of knowledge about mental disorders as well as through an imagined language to describe, measure, and compare diseases. This imagined universality was shaped by the social, cultural, and political milieu of the postwar period. It was based on scientists' wish to emancipate citizens of the world, who were devastated by war, and help them adapt during the postwar rehabilitation process. These scientists believed that the global burden of mental disorders should be investigated through collective effort. They sought to identify what diseases looked like and determine whether they were comparable across cultures. According to Fromm, "Just as there is *folie à deux*, there is *folie à millions*": "There are universal criteria for mental health which are valid for the human race as such, and according to which the state of health of each society can be judged."[27] As a friend of the head of the mental health unit of the WHO, G. Ronald Hargreaves (1908–1962), Fromm believed that a "criterion of mental health is not one of individual adjustment to a given social order, but a universal one, valid for all men."[28] In much the same way, scientists who proposed the International Social Psychiatry Project believed that the search for an international understanding of mental disorders and subsequent classification efforts were a project of emancipation.

This book, by looking at a specific WHO project, responds to a wide range of questions posed by historians of science, medicine, and technology. They include: Why did scientists once boldly assume that mental illnesses looked universally alike? What was the purpose of establishing universal criteria for mental disorders? What cultural milieu catalyzed such scientific efforts? How did researchers establish the profile of a mental disorder? How did they classify mental disorders worldwide? How did they remain internationalist idealists in a world that was still widely divided? Did they carry out their promise to create a common language for psychiatric science? What were their achievements and discontents? These questions require an analysis of a historical period, from the end of World War II to 1979, when chapter V was added to *ICD-9*.

Although this was not the first period of international collaboration, medical scientists managed, during these decades, to extend their scope across the Atlantic under the umbrella of the newly established United Nations. Their project was inspired by a thought-provoking concept—world citizenship. The concept is similar to "global citizenship," the transcendence of national borders that we talk about nowadays. However, "world citizenship" not only implies that the responsibilities and rights of individuals are derived from their humanity, but suggests that all human beings belong to a single race. This cutting-edge concept was coined in response to the devastation of World War II and the shared obligation for postwar rehabilitation. As Richard Horton, the editor-in-chief of *The Lancet*, elaborates in 2018: "If one views global health using this broader lens, the historical turn that was the decisive and creative moment for the birth of global health was surely decolonization. It was decolonization, beginning in the 1950s with legacies that continue to this day, which illuminated the myriad pressures that shape the health of peoples worldwide."[29]

Through the efforts of the WHO, medical scientists applied their view of an entire world composed of one human race with a common profile for mental disorders. Their efforts overlapped with decolonization, which gathered momentum toward the end of World War II. In the Anglo-American context, the project coincided with the growing trend to deinstitutionalize mentally ill patients from hospitals to the community.[30] More important, the WHO relied heavily on the contribution of its member states, particularly experts from developing or underdeveloped countries. In the end, the vision shared among WHO scientists promoted the feasibility of international mental health research, despite epistemic and practical criticisms and challenges. Nonetheless, international psychiatric epidemiology evolved to become a discipline that focuses both on numbers and on the form and content of suffering.

Problematizing the History of Global Health

The history of international social psychiatry is a lens through which to decipher the history of transnational medicine. Historians have, in general, been concerned with globalization, comparison, and transnational networks. They identify circumstances in which currency, commodity, and ideas develop a global reach, often as they undergo processes of conversion.[31] By contrast, at certain points, divergent processes may also lead to dissimilarity. In the history of medicine, diseases, concepts, disciplines, and institutions are principal areas of analysis. Medical historian Mark Harrison redefines the "global turn" in the historiography of medicine, noting that the original approach has had little substantial effect in the field. Citing examples from the past two centuries, he notes that much scholarship considers medical traditions within colonies or nation states. Harrison proposes a broader perspective, with a wider geographical range, looking at how "Western medicine" has emerged in the non-West, particularly through a global market that has allowed complex trajectories of disease transmission to develop in tandem with commodity exchange.[32] Trade, he argues, affects the global development of medicine.[33] Here I apply this insight to consider perspectives from the "non-West."

In the 1990s, transnational historians began to call for studies to look at the post-World War II foundational ideology underpinning the production of knowledge in important international organizations. The term "transnational history" has become popular over the past three decades. In that same period, scholars have argued for the importance of internationalizing history. Akira Iriye framed twentieth-century cultural internationalism as the exchange of ideas, cultures, and persons from various countries and agencies.[34] Glenda Sluga conceptualized the modern history of internationalism as an age of nationalism and national interests.[35] The decades after World War II are the most investigated period in global history. The war gave rise to technology that made possible the compression of space and time, and the postwar decades saw the emergence of a global society, the end of colonialism, and the specter of the Cold War.[36] This period was marked by the division of the world into new spheres of influence, the advent of new migration patterns, the growth of consumerism and the middle class, the establishment of new international relations and alliances, and the accelerated development of scientific theories. The actions of the WHO and the development of a discipline addressing mental health during this period are crucial to understanding the globalization of scientific trends.

Global health provides considerable opportunity to scrutinize historiographies. Here, I do not dwell on disputes over existing theories. Instead, I explore a less investigated but critical story. As Sunil Amrith notes, the twentieth century saw the internationalization of health, pursued by national institutions and international organizations and driven by purveyors of nationalist and internationalist ideologies.[37] The Office International d'Hygiène Publique (OIHP) based in Paris was the precursor of contemporary intragovernmental health organizations. With a permanent secretariat and a committee consisting of senior public health officials from member governments, it operated from 1908 to the advent of World War I. During the interwar period, a Health Organization was created under the League of Nations to "endeavour to take steps in matters of international concern for the prevention and control of disease."[38] Both OIHP and the Health Organization of the League of Nations were Euro-centered. After World War II, the design of the World Health Organization took a new direction. It not only incorporated public health scholars in the Americas, but it was also one of the many United Nations organizations that made a concerted effort at peacemaking and postwar economic rehabilitation.

From the late 1940s to the mid-1960s, the WHO's projects embodied the complexity of the period. Their story reflects the call of transnational historians to study organizations. Organizations like the WHO facilitated many aspects of globalization and provided a platform that allowed the economy, politics, culture, and ideology of one country to penetrate another. The end of World War II opened boundaries across nation states and created a platform to attract international attention to issues such as humanitarian relief, development, human rights, global health, and environmental conservation. International organizations are not the only players in transnational history, but they are the most important players in processes that transcend the interests of individual nations.[39] In establishing its postwar health-related agenda, the WHO occupied a position that can inform transnational historians as they consider the voices of marginalized people or groups. The unique structural design and legacy left behind by its precursor in the League of Nations, the vision shared among experts, and the realpolitik of the Cold War all contributed to new ways to tackle the global agenda of human health.[40]

The transnational history of medicine has focused mostly on infectious diseases, such as malaria, typhus, polio, dengue fever, and cholera, but several studies have addressed the transnationalization of psychiatric or psychological topics, although not in the postwar period. Ernst and Mueller review methodologically diverse historical studies to describe, interpret, and analyze psychiatric themes in Anglo-Saxon, Germanic, and Francophone European countries. Their work involves "systemic comparison, transfer, shared history, connected history, and *histoire croisée*."[41] They challenge and defy "ideologically and conceptually fraught terms such as medical 'system,' 'center' versus 'periphery,' 'eastern' versus 'western,' 'traditional' versus 'modern,' and even 'global' versus 'local.'"[42] The transnational approach, they explain, attempts to "reach beyond the conceptual and thematic confines of single-country case studies prevalent in most histories of psychiatry and mental health." Transnational analysis "take[s] issues with an a priori spatial focus on nation states with histories that take the boundaries of modern nations as their main reference point and framework of analysis" to "reify politically imposed borders and, in Benedict Anderson's sense, 'imagined communities.'"[43] Accounts comparing psychiatric systems across Europe, for example, trace and examine the key connections and scientific networks from which mental health practitioners in various nations (or nation states) take inspiration. The chapters on psychiatric history in non-Western countries, however, are incomplete. A volume edited by Roelcke et al. focuses on the crossing of geographical and linguistic boundaries and questions the so-called universalization of psychiatric subjects by investigating local variations in knowledge production.[44] The authors employ various methods to examine individual psychiatrists as narrative-constructing instruments, to track the shift in the attitudes of psychiatrists by citing quantitative studies, and to investigate the effect of psychiatrists' emigration on the field of psychiatry during the interwar period.

The transnational approach has become increasingly popular among historians and sociologists of psychiatric sciences, but the questions they ask and the problems they solve differ. The relationship between international organizations and the Global South remains a subordinate topic in most studies examining the postwar global health agenda. For the past few years, some historians have been endeavoring to write the history of transcultural psychiatry.[45] I have also worked with other historians of psychiatry to critique and consolidate existing historiography of psychiatry globally. We edited special issues to map out psychiatries worldwide and see how psychiatric theories and practices have been invented and reinvented through transnational professional networks and in less noticed regions.[46] Now, in this book, I am painting a bigger picture by not only analyzing the modus operandi of the WHO's mental health project but also exploring the role of experts participating in that project. Furthermore, I seek to analyze the "transnationality" of mental health through a case study of the interactions between the WHO and developing countries, and I explore the infrastructure of scientific knowledge production at various levels.

Moreover, I discuss the effect of postwar technology, reasoning with statistical methods, Cold War culture, and other social and cultural factors on these projects. Ultimately, I comment on the functions and limits of these projects and what they mean to modern psychiatry. By examining an institution, this book tells a story of scientists who were agents of knowledge and who managed to establish a scientific paradigm and produce a common scientific language in the process of post-World War II rehabilitation. I explore the ways in which these scientists interacted with the WHO's infrastructure, the ecology of their work, and the sea change in international relations of which they were a part.

The stories narrated here recount the theoretical debates and technical difficulties encountered by experts which, although they occurred half a century ago, still provide important background for today's agenda in these scholarly fields. They tell an institutional history in which earlier debates prove relevant to recent global mental health initiatives. Scholars today are still asking whether mental disorders share universal profiles, how symptoms of mental disorders are manifested in local contexts, and how psychiatric epidemiology and medical anthropology should inform each other to improve discourse among disciplines. In the past several decades, epidemiologists have attempted to answer these questions by refining their methods for data collection and analysis. Anthropologists have endeavored to reach less-known corners of the world, challenge norms, and piece together a broader picture of global mental health. But what they have not done is offer a perspective from which to understand how these questions emerged across countries over time, how they were tackled in a newly established international organization, and what obstacles and challenges analysts had to face.

The story presented in this book is a two-way approach to studying a history of the co-production of scientific knowledge: from the perspective of the WHO and from the perspective of its member states. Until now, few analysts have considered the WHO's role in the cross-national development of "world citizenship." Few recollect the time-consuming and labor-demanding task of statistics accomplished without computers. Few have attended to the story of Taiwan, a health entity currently not recognized by the United Nations, as the country entered the world health system and coordinated a complex, large-scale project. Yet, in the context of early postwar international relations, Taiwan represented the intricate relationship between international health organization and developing state. As one of the WHO's collaborating member states, Taiwan, also representing China, exemplified the ecology of work within the organization and its strategic bond with a developing country, albeit "an absurdity which is outstanding even in this era of absurdities," as its Director-General Brock Chisholm described Taiwan's representation of China.[47] Such absurdity, in the end, provides a benchmark for scholars of global health to speculate about the WHO's overly idealistic rationale. Although Taiwan's sociogeographic characteristics were ideal for most of the WHO's public health projects, the country had its own motives for wanting to join. Despite Taiwan's being used as a template for the WHO to test its rationale in underdeveloped countries, Taiwanese professionals aspired to be a part of international society. By looking at the limitation of the project and its evolution, I also examine the extent to which the contributions of collaborating member states made the WHO's project truly global.

Histories of the problem of classifying mental disorders—which typically highlight the peculiarity of the *DSM* system, stressing the epistemological turn between its second and third editions and the controversies between its fourth and fifth editions—tend to overlook the *ICD* system and its significance and accountability in global health governance.[48] Chapter V of *ICD-9* was the first classification of mental disorders produced by international collaboration and validated among the member states. This chapter also crystalized the WHO's health-for-all objective and the intellectual input of developing countries. The problems, difficulties, and disputes the WHO encountered during two decades of meticulous effort reflect those that continually appear in *ICD*'s reissuing process. On one hand, as an account that resonates with the social history of medicine, the story of the *ICD* complements the historical WHO narratives, which were written mostly in a conventional and chronological manner as institutional history.[49] On the other hand, the picture of international or global mental health is now one of hegemony, in which one system dominates.[50] Therefore, this book ironically echoes the demand made by historians of global health to decolonize the work of international health organizations and world standards.[51]

Moreover, responding to science studies, scholars are concerned about the social construction of scientific knowledge.[52] The story told in this book presents the WHO's efforts to make mental health count as a part of global health and as a formal science with its own methods, epistemology, and research agenda. Earlier science studies focused on laboratories and scientists' practices in lab settings. But in this book, I look at an institution in its idealistic and globalized cultural milieu. By examining a global network of experts who immersed themselves in transnational activities, I show how the WHO created useful knowledge in social psychiatry. Traveling the world, these experts established a network of like-minded researchers and practitioners who developed global social psychiatry and subsequent systems of international psychiatric classification.[53] With both national and international identities, they produced expertise that they applied differently at global and local levels. In addition to the globalized space, their work depended on the presence of nonhuman agents, namely the technology they used. The WHO's work was originally meant to be a bottom-up science-making endeavor that gathered local knowledge from around the world. However, its bureaucracy and the experts' desire to pursue "the international" had prevented the organization from carrying out this ideal.

The writing of this book relies heavily on archives I consulted over almost a decade of research and is based on the groundwork of my doctoral project. Primary sources include memoranda from the WHO's projects, minutes of meetings, conference proceedings, correspondence among scientists, and medical journal articles. Archives include the World Health Organization (Switzerland); the British Society of Psychoanalysis, the Institute of Psychiatry, the London School of Hygiene and Tropical Medicine, Queen Mary University of London, Wellcome Collection, the Bethlem Museum of the Mind, The National Archives, and King's College London (United Kingdom); and the Alan Mason Chesney Medical Archives of the Johns Hopkins Medical Institutions and the National Institutes of Health (United States).

An Overview of This Book

The chapters in this book are loosely arranged in chronological order. However, they are presented with a thematic approach to cover more comprehensively all aspects of the questions I explore. Readers who want an overview of the exact time of events can consult the timeline provided at the beginning of the book. Following this introduction, chapter 2, "Structure," explores the relationship between "world citizenship" and the birth of international social psychiatry. It examines the postwar conceptual turn in the research of mental disorders by looking at the role of the WHO in promoting international mental health. This initiative was a rehabilitative endeavor to help people face the psychological devastation of the postwar period. Toward the end of World War II, nation states and institutions began to seek "preparedness," to allow peace to endure and to prevent further atrocities. Psychiatrists, government planners, and postwar rehabilitation workers gradually saw mental disorders as a significant burden for urbanized societies. I thus start with "combat neurosis" among soldiers and their problematic homecoming and describe how the anxiety of contracting mental disorders spilled over from soldiers to civilians. The chapter focuses on the International Congress on Mental Health that took place in 1948, a bona fide "international" congress that claimed to be more functional than the WHO in discussing global issues under the shadow of the Cold War and the potential for international collaboration in science and medicine. The congress created the unit that still oversees issues of mental health at the WHO.

Topics in the Mental Health Unit of the WHO included global awareness of mental rehabilitation; strengthening the link between psychiatry and public health; and the idea of world citizenship in the era of large-scale, cross-cultural studies of mental health. "World citizenship," a term propagated by Brock Chisholm, the first director of the WHO, presumes the universality of humanity, together with the aspiration of promoting peace. These topics shaped the basis of the WHO's scientific practice and augmented the fields of psychiatry and public health, which then gave rise to a new paradigm of mental health at the international level—that is, psychiatric epidemiology. In chapter 2, I explore the long consideration of the so-called manageable project of international collaborative research, which was proposed by G. Ronald Hargreaves, the first head of the WHO's Mental Health Unit, and discuss a range of finished and unfinished works that were produced before large-scale, cross-cultural projects. I describe similar projects in various geographical areas from which the WHO eventually drew its "experts."

Chapter 3, "Method," looks at how a project on international social psychiatry was shaped by the WHO's early skeletal structure, and comments on methodology the organization developed in its first large-scale international study of mental health. Started in the mid-1960s, this International Social Psychiatry Project established the foundation of international mental health research. (In this book, I will use the term "International Social Psychiatry Project" to refer to the WHO's Ten-Year Plan in Psychiatric Epidemiology and Social Psychiatry, initiated in 1964. It is not a single project but a venture involving interconnecting subprojects, research centers, and collaboration among them.)[54] The chapter has three parts: the background of the project, its content, and its aftermath. Most outstanding were its renowned classification and standardization of psychiatric diseases and the pilot studies of schizophrenia through cross-cultural methods of assessment and diagnosis. Besides creating a common global language, the classification and pilot studies also created diagnostic methods, statistical procedures, and other useful instruments for future research. The results of the International Pilot Study of Schizophrenia (IPSS) convinced many people of the viability of international and cross-cultural research. They also seemed to confirm the presumptions that the founders of the WHO made about the "universal mind."

In chapter 4, "Experts," I explore how WHO-recruited scientists enabled the exchange of knowledge, sharing of methods, and formation of collaborative research between the organization and its member states. I first provide short examples in which knowledge transfer occurred between the WHO and its Latin American and African collaborators. In a more detailed case, I consider the factors that enabled the WHO to invite Tsung-yi Lin (1920–2010) from Taiwan to become its medical officer and head the social psychiatry project. Taiwan stands out as a curious case. It relished two decades of membership in the WHO until 1972, when the People's Republic of China took its place at the United Nations. Young and ambitious, Taiwan exported a model of knowledge production and a medical officer to Geneva to command the WHO's first several international social psychiatry projects. I examine the factors that catalyzed the link between the WHO and Taiwan's researchers, and I analyze the active and passive roles their studies played in postwar decolonization and scientific internationalism as the United Nations and its agencies created a new world order. Influenced by the survey-based Japanese ethnological studies in the first half of the twentieth century and designed to build a discipline after World War II, the epidemiological psychiatric research conducted in Taiwan not only reflected the vision of international scientific communities to "deracialize" the human sciences but also fulfilled the WHO's ideology of world citizenship.[55] This cultural determinism matched then-dominant neo-Freudian theories of psychopathology, which had moved away from the biodeterminism of colonial psychiatry. It also laid the foundation for establishing universal profiles of mental disorders.

Responding to existing historical accounts of the WHO's projects, this chapter also offers a conceptual framework for rethinking the relationship between Geneva and its target: developing countries. The tie between the WHO and its member states exemplifies and even goes beyond what science historians call a "trading zone"—that is, is a space for collaboration among scientists of various cultures, languages, and disciplines who mobilize by exchanging thoughts and methods. This collaboration also reflects the "dreamscape" propagated by science and technology studies, with developing countries shaping their identities with sociotechnological imagery beyond the WHO's Geneva-centered ideological framework.[56] The efforts of national self-fashioning and administrative pilgrimage enabled scientists from the WHO's member states to participate in international scientific projects. Though they were summoned from around the world, they mostly shared similar scientific training. The projects required a world mutually imagined by headquarters and member states. These scientists' activities corroborated recent scholarly discussions on the critical role technical experts could play in the movement of scientific knowledge across borders.[57] This short-lived optimism, however, promoted both achievements and fallacies.

Chapter 5, "Technology," presents the infrastructure of metrics and scientists' pursuit of technology. I depart, at least a bit, from institutional history to analyze a critical determinant in shaping the WHO's International Social Psychiatry Project. The chapter discusses scientists' obsession with standardization and their pursuit of a range of up-to-date technologies, both of which organized the WHO's "technological turn." Here I question the common imagery of a standardized world and technology-influenced knowledge-making, and I address a common query in the history of science: Can there be a revolutionary science or technology without corresponding revolutionary social change? Structural factors link social change to the legacy of war, to newly established internationalism, and to the formation of international health organizations. For the WHO, standardization of biomedical data among different member states was the first step toward international collaboration.

In the WHO's work on social psychiatry, the aim of standardization was not only to synchronize sectors in the organization but also to produce a common language of psychiatry. Standardization was thus both the reason for international collaboration and its desired product. Psychiatrists standardized their research methods by inventing interview instruments, unifying descriptions of symptoms, and developing statistical means to analyze and classify disease profiles. Such efforts could not have been conducted without advancements in technology during the decade. During the 1950s and 1960s, new forms of contemporary technology, whether used in industry or in the household, were being developed at an unprecedented pace. From scientists' expressions of wild hope to the execution of a project, investigators enjoyed the convenience of almost worldwide electric telegraph to communicate with each other. The investigators also discovered the capacity of videography to capture human affect. Although they had to wait for computing technology to facilitate the heavy work of calculation, they were able to develop software that met their needs.

In the sixth chapter, "Discontent," I analyze why the optimism of the International Social Psychiatry Project turned to dissatisfaction. Echoing current critiques of psychiatric epidemiology and the classification of mental disorders in global mental health, I use the concept of the "export processing zone" to reappraise the WHO's early modality for knowledge production. The WHO's ten-year International Social Psychiatry Project established a paradigm for international collaboration in mental health research by rewriting a better-received international disease classification system while also laying the foundation for further international epidemiological research. Chapter V of *ICD-9* provided a gold standard for psychiatrists in countries where mental health infrastructure was still underdeveloped. It laid the methodological groundwork for the Determinants of Outcome of Severe Mental Disorders (DOSMED) study of schizophrenia, another large-scale study that, with the collaboration of its twelve diverse sociocultural research sites, almost ratified a universal profile for functional mental disorder.[58] Placing the WHO's first projects on social psychiatry in the framework of historical and social studies of science raises questions about evaluating its overall effect, including its contribution to modern psychiatry, its significance in global development, and its representation of knowledge production. The complex links between the WHO and its member states describe an export processing zone, a relationship in which globalists in the headquarters and technocrats of science mutually imagine each other as enjoying an equal world citizenship. This relationship allows the possibility of a common scientific language and the capacity to apply it in the development of technologies, both to understand mental illnesses as a whole and to improve human welfare.

Finally, in the epilogue, I look at what this book's story might imply amid current debates in trans/cultural psychiatry and global mental health. Scientists have shifted their concerns from the creation of universal metrics to refocusing on the importance of local matrixes. The WHO's International Social Psychiatry Project excelled in ways scientists in the past could have neither imagined nor achieved. Some developing countries, however, voiced concerns about the WHO's intended beneficiaries. Skepticism grew when, upon completing its study on schizophrenia and attempting to broaden its inquiry to include such nonpsychotic disorders as depression, the WHO was unable to establish a universal profile for these disorders. Although they replicated research on many disorders, researchers never achieved consensus on the profile of any disorder other than schizophrenia. For example, anthropologists discovered that "depression" was not commonly expressed in China. Criticisms of the *ICD*, such as that it perpetuated category fallacies, thus began to emerge. Over time, other identifiable, culture-bound syndromes came to reflect the culturally sensitive autonomy of these countries, and new approaches and disciplines sought to tackle mental disorders worldwide. Many countries developed their own systems for disease classification, challenging the research paradigm established by the WHO and its efforts to improve epidemiology research.

Several years after the WHO's International Social Psychiatry Project, epidemiologists not only questioned the hypothesis and methodology of its original bold plan but also added nuance to the project's explanations of mental disorders as they gradually became a global burden on treatment and care. On one hand, in developing countries like China, a region entirely neglected by the WHO's early projects, psychiatrists held complex attitudes toward developing their own classification system and integration with the *ICD*. On the other hand, the WHO not only managed better integration with the *DSM* system, which was becoming influential internationally, but also sought a more concise and expedient classification and diagnostic system for adoption worldwide. The WHO then resorted to better epidemiological methods and more democratic ways of knowledge production by considering the views of experts from different disciplines as well as the opinions of patients. According to renowned psychiatrist Kenneth Kendler, classifying diagnoses of diseases can be seen as iteration, the mathematical metaphor used by historian of science Hasok Chang to describe temperatures.[59] In this book, however, with my limited training in clinical psychiatry, I showcase the WHO's International Social Psychiatry Project. I do not seek to redeem the work of these scientists but to reveal a process of psychiatric knowledge production that was contingent on a changing worldview, the transformation of world politics, a reliance on available technology, and debates among stakeholders of this large scientific enterprise.

As an account of the history of medicine and the making of scientific knowledge, this book stops short of pointing toward a direction for psychiatric epidemiology or disease classification. As a historian, I employ representative events to decipher the purpose of a concept and the knowledge-making project that it inspired. I show that this process of knowledge production was contingent on factors specific to time and place. In the end, I elucidate the significance of the WHO's early research agenda, its idealism and limitations, and its relationship to the perpetual challenges encountered in the long history of science.

2 Structure

After World War II, mental health slowly became a global issue. When most countries were attempting to recover from the war's damage, cross-national governance of health expanded far beyond that of prewar Europe, with the establishment of the World Health Organization in 1948. From the mid-nineteenth century to the interwar period, international sanitary conferences and the Health Office at the League of Nations had proved unable to incorporate countries outside major colonial trade routes. Not until the end of World War II did "international" health cross the Atlantic to reach the Americas. The "World" in "World Health Organization" thus reflected the internationalist world order envisioned by postwar idealists. At its beginning, the WHO was invigorated by the postwar euphoria and the growing spirit of internationalism among planners.[1] On the basis of this idealism, its research presumed a single human race and sought causes of psychiatric diseases that posed major threats to all humanity.

The attempt to internationalize the study of mental health hinged on the idea of "world citizenship." It was not a new idea, especially for the many postwar internationalists who served international organizations. In the field of mental health, however, it was Canadian psychiatrist Brock Chisholm (1896–1971), the first director general of the WHO, who managed to bring together the idea of world citizenship with the work of mental health. World citizenship presumes a universality of human minds, together with an unstated aspiration for enduring peace after the devastation of World War II.[2] It is a combination of ideology, social movement, and political aspiration that advocates for a basic set of rights that apply within and among nations. This ethos helped to shape scientific practices associated with the WHO, and served as the guiding principle that provided the basis for WHO projects to survive the Cold War. As a military psychiatrist from Canada, Chisholm had been notorious for his embrace of eugenics and his emphasis on the role of family in children's education. After World War II, however, his focus gravitated toward the belief that a healthy mental state, loosely defined as the absence of neurotic behaviors, could eliminate international conflict. He came to reflect on the causes of war and sought to investigate collective human neurosis.[3] Thus, he called for governments, not just members, to support the newly formed United Nations to combine "world health" and "world peace."[4]

Chisholm's utopian concept was cutting-edge but not unique; it was also shared by many other foresighted scientists who believed in addressing public health crises through research and planning. Applying the notion of world citizenship, psychiatrists extended the scope of concern for the effects of war trauma from veterans to global civilians. Their efforts eventually led to the WHO's International Social Psychiatry Project, the outcome of which was the foundation of subsequent epidemiological studies and the international classification of mental disorders. Drawing on the concept of world citizenship, psychiatry changed to incorporate two perspectives. One was the trauma of war and the need for postwar rehabilitation; the other was postwar decolonization and the prospect of world peace. Psychiatrists sought to understand mental illness internationally as the first step of a large-scale endeavor that, over time, would globalize mental health research. For its first three decades, starting as a small-scale initiative, the WHO sought to gather experts and funding and to develop methods to produce practical knowledge that would be useful for the expansion of mental health research at the international level. After 1970, the organization applied a technocratic approach to standard making and enforcement of norms, as its scientists began to apply a more empirical, knowledge-based methodology for developing health policies.[5] The shift to an empirically based psychiatry, however, depended on sufficiency of staff, availability of research methods, advancement of technology, and myriad other factors for facilitating a vast institutional enterprise in the shadow of the Cold War.

The idea of world citizenship was closely related to the then-popular sentiment of scientific internationalism. There are different ways to account for the origins of scientific internationalism. From one perspective, from the end of the nineteenth century to the advent of World War II, the scientific community had grown increasingly diverse, while simultaneously, international scientific organizations had begun to proliferate. Needing to accommodate the highly heterogeneous backgrounds of scientists, these international organizations set communication as their first goal, and this goal catalyzed a wide range of work that focused on the universalities of scientific knowledge.[6] From another perspective, the ethos of scientific internationalism—the idea that scientific cooperation among governments could contribute to broader goals of promoting international peace and prosperity—inspired organizations such as the Health Organization of the League of Nations and the WHO to incorporate various health-related topics into what we now understand as global health. Scientific internationalism had also existed during the interwar period. According to historian Glenda Sluga, the foundation of "objective facts," such as steam, electricity, trade, and the novelty of international organizations, served as the basis of this ideology, causing the "international turn" for historians to plow through a wider range of contexts beyond the national level.[7] In the realm of science, advances in genetic research and a belief in biological integration triggered optimistic assumptions about universal scientific knowledge, which transcended national boundaries and loyalties.[8] This knowledge could be produced through cross-national research cooperation and information sharing. Despite its hopefulness, however, scientific internationalism, in the era shortly before and after World War II, became a political instrument exploited by different states to serve national interests and policies.[9]

Speaking of scientific internationalism after World War II, Akira Iriye used the term "cultural internationalism" to refer to the vision of the world order that developed in response to the growth of nationalism around the world in the late nineteenth century. Under this ideology, the best way to maintain global political stability is to undercut the appeal of nationalism by bringing different cultures into contact. By generating mutual understanding and recognition of shared humanity, war could be avoided.[10] This innovation had been envisaged by various national governments but required the creation of the United Nations, which promoted scientific internationalism through the Food and Agriculture Organization, the International Labour Organization, and the United Nations Educational, Scientific, and Cultural Organization (UNESCO). For example, the first director of UNESCO, Julian Huxley (1887–1975), who served from 1946 to 1948, made explicit the organization's commitment to "some form of world political unity, whether through a single world government or otherwise, as the only certain means for avoiding war."[11] UNESCO has been facilitating the creation and propagation of scientific and humanistic knowledge ever since.

The story presented in this book looks at the work of the WHO and a group of visionary thinkers within and outside the organization who have also been striving toward "a shared commitment to achieve better health for everyone, everywhere," as stated nowadays.[12] This ethos was reflected in the San Francisco meeting that took place in 1946, where the word "world" was deliberately placed in the name of the organization to reflect a spirit that would include developed and underdeveloped countries and those that were still colonies.[13] In the immediate postwar period, the WHO's founders identified research agendas, created norms and standards, and produced evidence-based data to provide technical support to improve the mental health of all humankind. The organization's proposal to augment public health with mental health further facilitated the effort to establish and classify universal profiles of mental disorders. This ethos gave birth to the WHO's social psychiatry project. Yet it represented an optimism for global health that was too good to be true. The project facilitated collaboration among psychiatrists and social scientists to establish a new science, a new language, and a new paradigm for understanding the human mind. Though fueled by the idealism of scientific internationalism, the project also faced challenges. The story of the WHO's social psychiatry project, therefore, can tell us much about the difficulty of conducting global mental health research.[14]

Lessons of War

Warfare has profoundly influenced psychiatry. Historians of psychiatry have written a range of theoretical accounts regarding the origin and transformation of traumatic psychologies. One of the most discussed is a condition of war-related trauma variously known as "shell shock," "combat exhaustion," or "war neurosis." These military psychiatric categories stemmed mainly from the two world wars and later from the United States Vietnam War, which gave rise to "posttraumatic stress disorder," first included in the *DSM* classification system in 1980. Historians and anthropologists have discussed at length changing disease terminology and the influence of warfare on psychiatric disciplines. During the interwar period, an increasing number of specialized institutions were established to provide treatment for traumatized soldiers.[15] Shell shock, however, was never deemed a public health issue that burdened the state resources. At the international level, it hardly registered as a general concern. Before and during World War II, battlefield disorders were still causally linked to individual capacities affected by external stimulation. Research during World War II sought to uncover the role of draftees' socioeconomic status on mental capacity at the frontline. For example, US psychologists studied the incidence and types of mental disorder among 60,000 Boston-area draftees to catalog factors contributing to the mental health of draft-age men.[16]

After World War II, a group of neo-Freudian psychiatrists, predominantly in the United States, began to apply relational approaches to psychoanalysis and psychotherapy to war-related conditions. Their theories marked a break from German or French psychiatric traditions before and during the war. Instead of looking at the internal drive in human beings to thrive despite a harsh environment, they shifted their focus to the individual's search for comfort and safety.[17] In doing so, they had to study factors external to the human body that influenced the sense of security. For example, *Men under Stress* (1945), written by Roy Grinker (1900–1993) and John Spiegel (1911–1991), was a classic example of how the recognition of combat stress among returning soldiers was popularized in American society.[18] In addition, the US military psychiatrist Harry Stack Sullivan (1892–1949), who believed social and cultural forces were responsible for mental illnesses, reframed psychopathology as interactional rather than intrapsychic. He thus reconceptualized Freudian theory to situate interpersonal factors and personality development as the source of breakdown among soldiers.[19] Extending psychoanalytic theories to encompass social and cultural influence not only broke with Freudian tradition but also severed the human mind from its biological assumptions. Mental disorders now became "social."

New explanations for causes of war-related mental disorders also spurred psychiatrists to consider whether these mental breakdowns were preventable in the military context. Several British and US psychiatrists, for example, attempted to produce a psychiatry that could prepare individuals and communities for adverse experiences, and, beginning in the interwar period, prevention of mental suffering among soldiers took precedence over treatment.[20] Novel treatments for shell shock were endorsed by new institutions, such as Cassel Hospital in Kent and Tavistock Clinic, now in West Hampstead, London. New theories were developed to negotiate between behaviorism and Freudian psychoanalysis. Even as some lessons of war were forgotten during peacetime, individuals continued to probe the aftermath of the Great War.

During World War II, British and US psychiatrists tacitly agreed to undertake preventive psychiatry by screening soldiers' intelligence and personalities. The screening ensured that only soldiers who were both physically strong and mentally robust were sent to the front line. For example, in his monograph on the shaping of psychiatry by war, a British military psychiatrist based at the Tavistock Clinic emphasized the quality of men: "the job of the army is to evaluate these [men] and modify as many as possible for preventing breakdown. When prevention fails, we must organize the most effective and rapid treatment."[21] G. Ronald Hargreaves, another Tavistock-trained military psychiatrist, who later became the head of WHO's Mental Health Unit, established Progressive Matrices, a kit for rapidly testing soldiers' intelligence. In the 1940s, Harry Stack Sullivan worked with the US Army Selective Service to develop a method for screening the personality types of military recruits to spare weak or unfit men from frontline duty. Rather than protect the healthy from mental breakdowns, these methods aimed to sort out potential victims of battlefield trauma.[22]

This focus on preventing mental disorders began to spill over to civilians. But such a move was not at first fully supported by psychiatric professionals, as they were torn between maintaining citizens' morale and more humanist approaches to mental well-being. In the wake of postwar devastation, medical practitioners began to draw their own conclusions about the human condition. Psychiatry promised explanations based on science. For example, as the head of the Medical Sciences Division of the Rockefeller Foundation, Alan Gregg (1890–1957) considered "the greatest unpleasant surprise of the war for medical men ... the importance of psychiatry and psychology."[23] Asked by Chisholm to chart the direction of mental health work in preparation for the International Congress on Mental Health, British child psychiatrist Kenneth Soddy (1911–1986), who led the Child Guidance Clinic and later founded the Children and Adolescent Psychiatric Department at the University College Hospital in London, made prevention, not treatment, the priority.[24] During the war, as head of the Canadian Army Medical Services, Chisholm noted the war's psychological effects.[25] Later, he deemed the postwar human condition a "valid" and "free-floating anxiety," which was "not necessarily seen to belong to its real source, but maybe just felt as a discomfort and unhappiness, a fear that 'something is wrong.'"[26] To Chisholm, responding to this minor anxiety would prevent major psychiatric disorders among the general population.

Toward the end of the war, however, psychiatrists were divided over whether the scrutiny applied to military recruits should be directed at civilians as well. From the perspective of the state, building sound and resilient citizens, ready for adversity, was important. But relief from the devastation of war was also a pressing issue. Treating civilians like soldiers now became a huge controversy. In the UK, psychiatrists at the Tavistock Clinic debated the appropriateness of employing nontherapeutic means on civilians in peacetime. For example, Edward Glover (1888–1972), influential for combining psychotherapy and criminology, opposed the military approach and questioned its feasibility, but he was unfortunately expelled from the British Psychanalytic Society for diverging from his colleagues who were ready to apply military approaches to civilians.[27] In the immediate postwar period, psychiatrists had not yet derived feasible methods of inquiry, apart from stressing the importance of mental health research for civilians.

After the war, a transient general concern arose about soldiers who fell mentally or neurologically ill. The film *Let There Be Light* (1946), by Hollywood director John Huston, documented a group of returning soldiers suffering from "battle fatigue" at Mason General Hospital in Long Island, New York. However, in an effort to quell anxieties and ensure the mental stability of veterans during the Cold War, the Army banned the documentary from public screening and commercial circulation until 1980.[28] Even within the profession, psychiatrists' attitudes toward techniques developed during the war were paradoxical. On one hand, the increase in mental disorders exposed by wartime screening caused anxiety among civilians.[29] On the other, psychiatrists were eager to exercise their newly acquired ability to assist those in need of psychiatric help.[30] For example, Karl Bowman (1888–1973), then president of the American Psychiatric Association (APA), asserted in his inaugural speech in 1946, "We believe that there is a science of human behavior; that it is possible to understand the causes of good and bad adjustment."[31] War devastation, however, had disrupted the scientific community and obstructed progress. In response, another APA president, Donald Ewen Cameron (1901–1967), reflected, "we live in a world where massive displacement and sudden death are strangers to no one, a world in which the continuous safety of the whole depends upon the goodwill of every part, but a world still tragically far from unity."[32] The anxiety of these psychiatrists paved a clear path for the development of mental health practices that focused on those outside the theater of war.

Mental Health as Public Health

Mental health professionals expressed distinctly new concerns during the postwar period. Their anxiety was immense and their initiatives many, but the concept of world citizenship eventually provided their core philosophy. Throughout its history, as Michel Foucault has argued, psychiatry has been used as an instrument to control the social order. Nonetheless, postwar internationalists were less likely to use it for this purpose. Instead, they developed a new form of psychiatry to address the burden of mental illness for individuals and communities. Its goal was to understand why certain people were particularly at risk for certain mental symptoms. Mushrooming psychiatric research aimed to identify stressors, risk factors, and other psychosocial contributors to mental illnesses. For the first time, the mental health agenda became a part of the two-century-old public health movement. Implementing mental health research and policies on an international scale, however, was still beset with difficulties.

Clinicians previously employed by the military dominated the field of international health,[33] and mental health was no exception. A number of eminent psychiatrists in international health organizations were military psychiatrists. For example, Jack Rawlings Rees (1890–1969) was the medical officer in the UK's Royal Army Medical Corps during the interwar period. Later trained at the Tavistock Clinic, he became its medical director in 1933.[34] Toward the end of World War II, he was charged with the care of Hitler's deputy, Rudolf Hess, then being held in a secret prison in Scotland. In 1948, Rees became the first chief organizer of the World Federation for Mental Health. Like Rees, Hargreaves worked for the Royal Army Medical Corps and during World War II implemented selection procedures and studied war-related neuroses. His study of men who evidenced no predisposition to mental breakdowns showed that they were still at risk of developing psychoneuroses, indicating the limitations of selective recruiting and pointing to the universality of mental disorders.[35]

The man who set the tone for world health, Brock Chisholm, was acclaimed in the 1930s for his pioneering ideas about preventive medicine and children's education as well as for his controversial endorsement of birth control, voluntary sterilization, eugenics, euthanasia, and masturbation. Before his epoch-making contribution to scientific practice, Chisholm's central concern had been human conflict. He had pondered the causes of conflict, its effects, and what psychiatrists could do to help people avoid further devastation. In 1945, Harry Stack Sullivan invited Chisholm to lecture on "The Psychiatry of Enduring Peace and Social Progress" at the William Alanson White Foundation, one of the most important training institutions for US psychoanalysts. In 1946, Sullivan published the lecture in *Psychiatry: Interpersonal Processes*, the journal he had founded in 1938, and it attracted feedback from numerous individuals and professional societies.[36] In response, readers even sent Chisholm their own proposals for psychiatric investigation.

Recognizing his own popularity, Chisholm extended his focus beyond the military. Either by invitation or on his own initiative, he contributed articles not only to academic journals but also to popular magazines. For example, he wrote "What Can I Do at Home about War or Peace?" for *Better Homes and Gardens*.[37] His prescription for the world community evoked both appreciation and controversy. Notable was his assertion that human beings shared a common destiny. In contrast, his attacks on traditional morality and what he considered superstition irritated religious groups. In 1951, Chisholm even announced that he was going to present the case of Santa Claus before the United Nations as a measure to disenchant local fictions and promote universal spirit.[38] "The man who killed Santa Claus" later proposed a prescription for world peace in 1953, after he had stepped down as the director general of the WHO. During his tenure, he had successfully managed several epidemics, including cholera outbreaks in Egypt and malaria in Greece and Sardinia. But he had remained relatively quiescent regarding psychiatry.

Chisholm's grand proposal for "Enduring Peace and Social Progress" matched similar views propagated by like-minded psychiatrists. He turned to humanism and world government. If individuals could come to their senses and learn to think and act globally, he reasoned, they would form a single human race, embodying world citizenship. During his term as the WHO's director general, Chisolm promoted collaborative work among nations, which he regarded as essential for the very survival of the race.[39] Earlier in 1948, the president of the APA, Winfred Overholser (1892–1964), had asserted the need to augment the principle of mental hygiene with the spirit of world citizenship as part of the pressing postwar mental health agenda: "With international tensions mounting there is an urgent need for the application of mental hygiene principles and for the concentration of the wisdom of all toward the practical application of psychiatry to the problems of world citizenship."[40] William Menninger (1899–1966), Overholser's successor at the APA, shared this view, emphasizing that psychiatric problems among civilians were directly related to the experience of war. A response, he suggested, should acknowledge "the prominence achieved by psychiatry in the military service, the education of the public because of the extensiveness of psychiatric casualties, the increased demands on all of us for [psychiatric] services."[41] But Menninger questioned whether psychiatry could effectively respond to an extensive, long-term demand, asking, "Do we have so many sub-specialties in psychiatry that we have inadequate knowledge of others than our own? Are we still too lacking in a basic set of agreements and tested knowledge and clinical methods so that we simulate each other's emotion more than intellection?"[42] Despite these doubts, Menninger had earlier, in 1946, persuaded President Harry Truman to sign a mental health law to provide research, prevention, diagnosis, and treatment for the mentally ill.[43]

The project that made world citizenship a feasible psychiatric premise began in 1953, the year Queen Elizabeth II was crowned in Westminster Abbey and Dwight Eisenhower was sworn in as US president. Society had become quite different from the period of "pactomania"[44] immediately after the war. Cars were hitting the roads in most cities; televisions began to appear in households. At the end of that year, Ronald Hargreaves, then in his fifth year as chief of the Mental Health Section of the WHO, delivered a paper, "Mental Hygiene and the Epidemiology of Psychiatric Disorders," at the Seminar on the Mental Health of the Eastern Mediterranean Region. His paper emphasized the need to develop psychiatric care outside asylums and to foster cooperation between public health and psychiatry personnel to promote prevention. Recognizing that some psychiatric disorders (e.g., schizophrenia) might include genetic factors, he hypothesized that full-blown disorders might develop only in the presence of various stressors. Hargreaves suggested, "These stressful experiences ... are not those which are unusual or exceptionally catastrophic, they are, on the contrary, those which are usual, and which are the common lot of all human beings." Hargreaves was referring not to devastation caused by human atrocities and natural disasters but to everyday stresses, such as work, parenting, schooling, and even weaning of infants.[45] His words acknowledged human universality and the need for mental health professionals to probe the causes of mental health issues.

After the 1953 seminar, the spirit of psychiatry shifted, and new research methods began to take shape. Psychiatrists now endeavored to combine the principle of social psychiatry with comparative measures, and to escalate it to the international level. In Buenos Aires, in 1953, Hargreaves delivered another paper, "Preliminary Statement on a Research Project Dealing with Mental Health and Disease from a Comparative Point of View," stating that researchers should apply comparative studies to human groups that are similar in most respects to explore the etiology of mental disorders. He was confident about this approach in part because such work had already been preceded by several attempts over the previous half century:

> Kraepelin's paper on comparative psychiatry formulated the problem at the beginning of the century, and the Milbank Memorial Fund's Symposium on the Epidemiology of Mental Disorder gives us an example of the current application of the method. It must be said, however, that the subject has so far not been dealt with in a truly systematic way, the reason for this being in all likelihood that it was until now practically impossible to carry it out in sufficient scope.[46]

Hargreaves referred to the "urgency" of pursuing this project "in the near future." He further proposed "[the] initial task of assembling the available evidence, collecting additional facts as seem necessary for securing the over-all usefulness of the existing material and of organizing the sum of our present knowledge with a view towards making truly systematic research possible."[47] He used the phrase "a manageable project" to describe a study that was necessary and practical to carry out for scholars worldwide who were immediately willing and able to participate in. He sought to resurrect Emil Kraepelin's early attempt at scientific psychiatric research, which presented the environmental, social, cultural, and ethnic factors that influenced the types, prevalence, and expression of mental illness.[48]

In modern psychiatry, Emil Kraepelin (1856–1926) has always been deemed the father of biological psychiatry. He strongly objected to then-popular Freudian theories and complained that psychoanalysis was unscientific.[49] That said, in addition to his anatomical research into the human brain, his extensive fieldwork crucially shaped modern survey methods in psychiatry. In 1904, Kraepelin had conducted a comparative survey of residents of the islands of Java in the colonial Dutch East Indies. Soon after, he developed an evidence-based, simple, and homogeneous nosology of psychotic disorders that had great impact on clinical psychiatry.[50] Although colored with the characteristics of racial science, Kraepelin's work was the contemporary prototype of cross-cultural psychiatric research. Hargreaves, however, later proposed an international effort, an epidemiological study that would promote future research and the greater good. He presented his project in his book *Psychiatry and the Public Health,* published in 1958, which defined psychiatric illnesses as diseases, much like cholera.[51] The project became a cornerstone of public health. Nevertheless, Hargreaves had to wait for more than a decade before his visionary project was carried out.

The WHO Model and Early Efforts in Mental Health

The globalization of modern psychiatry during the postwar period occurred in tandem with the development of international organizations, of which the WHO was a main player. Unlike its predecessors, such as the pre-World War I Office International d'Hygiène Publique and the Health Organization of the League of Nations during the interwar period, the WHO did not limit its scope to Europe but covered six regions worldwide. It and other UN agencies were based on the "spill-over" theory, endorsed by functionalist economists, such as David Mitrany (1888–1975), who proposed that international cooperation was the ideal measure to reduce antagonisms in the international environment.[52] Spill-over theorists stated that alleviating health challenges in less-developed countries would decrease conflict between states by equalizing resource distribution, which would then foster stability and facilitate world peace.

Health became an essential element in the Charter of the United Nations. In Article 55, the UN was meant to create the "stability and well-being which are necessary for peaceful and friendly relations among nations."[53] Its principle of "equal rights and "self-determination of peoples" pointed to the decolonizing nature of the new intergovernmental organization and its specialized agencies. The WHO was inaugurated on April 7, 1948, to achieve "the attainment by all peoples of the highest possible level of health." Its constitution drafted earlier in 1946 in San Francisco stated that "health is a state of complete physical, mental and social well-being and not merely the absence of disease or infirmity."[54] This was the first time mental health received attention as part of a global health agenda. At the WHO's subsequent

First World Health Assembly, held in Geneva, health professionals identified issues requiring urgent postwar rehabilitation. While mental health, however, was officially listed in the WHO's inaugural constitution only in 1948, it was not discussed until later at another congress organized outside of the organization.

The WHO had a unique structure and modus operandi. One aspect of its design was the decentralization of power in six regional offices. Against the backdrop of continuing colonialism, the African regional office was the sixth and final one to be created, after a delay. Another unique aspect of the WHO was that it ensured that recommendations issued from headquarters were distributed effectively. The decentralized design was intended to keep the WHO from becoming a "supranational organization." It was to remain an "instrument only," which would "take its instructions from the governments of the world, and for its personnel to do exactly as they were told to do by the people of the world through their governments."[55] In addition, the organization adopted a framework of "technical assistance." While transferring knowledge of science and technology, such a framework was meant to be purely instrumental without imposing Western countries' economic or political interests.[56] During the Cold War, even though the WHO was also enmeshed in the politics of the United Nations, it managed to incorporate participants from different parts of the world and stayed as neutral as it could.[57]

To enable its effective functioning, the WHO employed thematic projects or programs of advisory services, facilitated by expert advisory panels and committees. Advisories were important because the WHO was not intended to become a research center that had to hire its own in-house researchers. The operational style of the advisory services was never simple, though. To meet a country's request, a regional director would consult with national authorities to determine the type of international assistance needed. The WHO would then recruit a suitable expert or team and brief participants on the purpose of the project, the conditions in the region and country, and the administrative and technical procedures that the organization had found useful in similar circumstances. The regional office would assist with the necessary liaison and coordination with national counterparts and local services appointed to work with the expert or team.[58] Although declaring itself decentralized, WHO operations relied on a vertical organizational model.[59] The model was best exemplified, later in the mid-1950s, by the case of the

Malaria Eradication Program regarding the use of DDT and the principle of technical assistance in developing countries, despite that project's contentious achievements.[60] According to the original structural design of WHO, experts recruited from all over the world gathered at the Geneva headquarters, where they ran study groups and technical meetings, either as large conferences or small seminars, and concluded their discussions with technical reports. The reports, which were referenced by member states, provided authoritative direction for WHO policies and programs.

The 1948 International Congress on Mental Health

The WHO provided a hub for health professionals worldwide to meet, exchange ideas, and promulgate proposals. Its idealistic ambitions, however, dwindled within two years of its inaugural constitution. Much of the reason was its inevitable involvement in the heightening tension between superpowers and in the subsequent Cold War before the death of Joseph Stalin.[61] The organization could neither accommodate the participation of all nations nor prioritize mental health. But in 1948, mental health gained international attention in its own right when the International Congress on Mental Health played a pivotal role in facilitating international mental health research as an instrument for global rehabilitation. This phenomenon led to the establishment of the Expert Committee of the Mental Health Unit within the WHO and the birth of another organization, the World Federation for Mental Health (WFMH). These new organizations were expected to work together to promote international collaboration among mental health professionals; the former focused on international planning and the latter on local input.

The International Congress on Mental Health was organized by Michael Harvard of the National Association of Mental Health in the UK and was chaired by Jack Rawlings Rees, the head of psychiatric services in the British Army. Founded in 1946, the National Association of Mental Health was a nongovernmental organization and later became the currently renowned British charity Mind. The association took more than a year to plan, promote, and invite delegates to participate in the congress. In May, while the WHO was still an interim commission, Brock Chisholm was already promoting its role in mental health planning across the Atlantic. In a speech in New York, he expressed excitement about the upcoming congress: "Perhaps never before in history has there been a more important meeting of any kind than that Congress can be, if all the people qualified and obligated to attend, do so, and if they can at the same time ignore all sectional interest, all local or national loyalties, all matters of personal or individual prestige or advantage, and by a free pooling of their knowledge and experience, offer even a little, but concrete hope for a frightened world."[62] This statement was printed on a flyer circulated at the congress the following year.

By the time the WHO was officially established in Geneva in 1948, its membership policy allowed only member countries of the United Nations to join the organization—a provision that contradicted the idealism of its constitution, which advocated the idea of the highest attainable level of health for all people. Then Britain discouraged its own delegates from attending international conferences organized by bodies other than the WHO.[63] Nonetheless, Michael Harvard strategically attempted to gather delegates by issuing invitations to the congress through Britain's Foreign Office and by accepting personal applications. He intended to create a representative assembly of world citizens unhindered by the WHO's membership policy or by Cold War politics. For example, Germany, Japan, and Spain were initially banned by British law from attending the congress because the gathering was regarded as a British diplomatic mission,[64] but after their individual applications, these nations were allowed to attend. Soviet law, however, prevented that nation from sending a representative.

Understandably, during the immediate postwar period, the enterprise of mental health was not monopolized by psychiatrists or physicians. During the week of the International Congress, psychiatrists, anthropologists, and sociologists all gathered to search for "a basis for common human aspiration" regarding mental health. The congress was held at Central Hall in the City of Westminster, London, from August 16 to 21, 1948. The joining fee was only six British pounds. The weeklong conference was one of the few truly open-minded, cross-disciplinary invitational meetings that evoked an almost utopian vision within the field of mental health. The congress was composed of three conferences on child psychiatry, medical psychology, and mental hygiene. The agenda attested to the ambiguous attitudes among professionals toward mental illness. To achieve the goal of cultivating a sound mind in modern people, they were torn between the importance of family and the pursuit of liberal and democratic life. To fulfill the latter, delegates pointed out, large-scale rationalized methods were needed that surpassed the power of states.[65]

Despite conflicting ideas within the mental health community, the congress did arrive at some consensus. Its statement provided a rare example of international organizations collectively reflecting on the wrongdoing of modern science after World War II, asserting that "Few societies of which we have knowledge are wholly free from distortion of human impulse, sometimes on a large scale, such as racial oppression, or industrial conflict."[66] Scientists, its members explained, were compelled to face the dreadful "possibilities of biological and atomic warfare" because of "profound disquiet following two world wars, and the fear of a third catastrophe." Instead of initiating social reforms, the congress was determined to "infuse a scientific spirit into the movements of reform and reconstruction" in countries that suffered from the most recent war. The congress concluded with three main objectives related to recruiting specialists and suggestions for the newly founded UN specialized agencies:

1. To bring together representatives of the professions for the promotion of human well-being, with the aim of defining those conditions that will enable every man, woman, and child to develop full worth and dignity.
2. To bring suggestions to the notice of the United Nations' specialized agencies, for example, the United Nations' Educational, Scientific and Cultural Organization, whose objectives are relevant to the congress's theme, and the World Health Organization, which already accepts social, mental, and physical health as one and indivisible.
3. To encourage ever-widening activities of organizations concerned with mental health in many countries, having regard for different societies readiness to understand and accept new knowledge and methods of communication, from the most concrete to the most general.

Two new organizations related to mental health were in line with the congress's proposals: the Mental Health Expert Committee at the WHO and the World Federation of Mental Health. The former sought to foster international mental health; the latter replaced the International Committee for Mental Hygiene, the organization initiated by Clifford Beers (1876–1943), who, during the interwar period, was famously devoted to the "protection of the insane."[67] The Mental Health Expert Committee was expected to handle international surveys and develop international standards regarding research methodology. The WFMH would assess the universality of the Congress's statement from the viewpoints of various nations and cultures and suggest modifications for its improvement. WFMH leaders hoped it could divert psychiatrists away from the "psychiatric imperialism" that attempted to impose Western standards of behavior on other cultures, including the ways mental disorders were assessed and treated.[68] One of the first architects of the WFMH was Margaret Mead (1901–1978), who was by that time a celebrated anthropologist renowned for her books *Coming of Age in Samoa* (1928) and *Growing Up in New Guinea* (1930), based on her fieldwork in the South Pacific. Collaborating with UNESCO, Mead offered anthropological input, but unlike the WHO's vertical model, her project collected and disseminated knowledge of various cultures "with respect for their cultural values to ensure the social progress of the people."[69] WFMH records indicate that various experts maintained close correspondence with one another and were actively involved in meetings and study groups organized by both official bodies.

Although the practical considerations of these new international organizations were complex, the core agenda of the 1948 International Congress was simple: to treat minds damaged by war and develop methods of peacemaking by enhancing mental health. Its summary text, *Mental Health and World Citizenship*, asked several questions: "Can the catastrophe of a third world war be averted? Can the peoples of the world learn to cooperate for the good of all? On what basis is there hope for enduring peace?"[70] The postwar development of world psychiatry was, at least in part, rooted in these bold if rather naïve questions. Regardless of the lack of concrete measures to answer these questions, the prototype of social psychiatry research at the international level was gradually taking shape.

From "Collection of Hunches" to Practice of Collaboration

Around 1948, those first involved in international mental health had a consistent level of awareness regarding the relevant issues. During its first ten years, however, experts in the WHO never reached consensus about development priorities. Compared with other specialties, mental health encountered enormous challenges regarding the "extreme difference in the level and scope of development of treatment facilities, for all types of psychological disorder in different countries."[71] Thus, before a large-scale, systematic approach was completely formulated, the concerns of early visionaries about mental health, though diverse, had to be aligned. Theories and protocols were proposed to address the etiology of mental illnesses and to answer the question, "Why do human beings develop psychiatric symptoms?" The experts' concern shifted the direction of mental health beyond the desire to prevent mental deterioration from exposure to extreme experiences to the exploration of stressors encountered during human development. The focus thus shifted from removing mentally ill people from society to a community-oriented preventive psychiatry.

Now mental health professionals at the WHO realized that, before they could initiate preventive work, they needed to understand mental health problems across different nations. A unified understanding of mental disorders was thought to be the foundation needed for the WHO to further their research. Despite similar attitudes toward international collaboration, however, they lacked a useful methodology. And although WHO director Brock Chisholm recognized the importance of "learning from each other," he did not propose substantial practical methods to facilitate international work on mental health. Rather, his contributions were limited to random observations of selected populations and the identification of characteristic human emotions, such as anxiety and aggression.[72] In fact, the WHO listed mental health fifth among the most important postwar priorities in 1948. Several factors accounted for the delayed programming for mental health. First, categories like malaria and other endemoepidemic diseases were deemed more urgent, together with the administration of public health.[73] Another influential factor was Chisholm's status as a psychiatrist, which required distancing himself from prioritizing mental issues so that he would be perceived as neutral.[74] Although the committee was sluggish in its actions, it never stopped looking for urgent issues and assessing the immediate needs of society.

The WHO's Mental Health Expert Committee was drawn from an advisory panel of nearly a hundred members in thirty-eight countries. The members met for the first time in 1949 and carefully considered the principles that should govern the WHO's future activities regarding mental health. The committee's first session involved Antônio Carlos Pacheco e Silva from Brazil, Joseph Hadlik from Czechoslovakia, Yü-Lin Ch'eng from China, M. V. Govindaswamy from India, D. F. Rodger from Britain, G. Ronald Hargreaves also from Britain, and from the United States, William C. Menninger, who chaired the session. All were educated in France, Britain, and the United States, apart from Ch'eng, who was trained at Peking Union Medical

College, a medical school established by physicians closely affiliated with the Rockefeller Foundation and Johns Hopkins University.[75] They all shared the vision that emphasized preventive measures. The committee laid down principles that clearly reflected the new imperatives of mental health in the postwar era. First, they aimed to bolster preventive mental health by encouraging training and specialization in mental hygiene. Second, they were concerned about developing therapeutic and preventive psychiatric services for children. Finally, they saw the need to integrate mental health with other WHO activities, such as public health administration, maternal and child health, and nursing. In its first decade, the WHO assisted in the development of psychiatric services by making available qualified short-term consultants to help member states in law, hospital treatment, and personnel training. Apart from its own areas of focus, the Expert Committee was expected to work with other specialized agencies affiliated with the United Nations.

New Issues in Mental Health after World War II

Issues thrashed out by the WHO's Mental Health Expert Committee covered a wide range of topics, reflecting the emergent psychological needs of people overwhelmed by the Second World War. They also registered the common anxiety of humans facing a drastically changing world. But not all issues were persistent or far-reaching enough to gain the attention of all member states. Rather, the issues chosen reflected the early visions of the experts and echoed the priorities of the WHO or the United Nations. Most of the agenda items were discussed in study groups; some were dropped, whereas others became important projects. These choices could not be detached from the turmoil of international politics in the postwar world, which broadly influenced the WHO's altruistic philosophy. As table 2.1 illustrates, the Expert Committee's early technical reports reflected an activist postwar response to a pressing agenda in mental health. The themes discussed by the Expert Committee, however, were gradually narrowed down to several important topics; among more than three hundred technical reports produced by the WHO, including official Expert Committee and special study group reports, only eighteen were related to mental health.

Children became the WHO's main focus in mental health. Following the devastation of war, children left without caregivers experienced

Table 2.1
Mental health themes of WHO's Technical Report Series and Study Group Reports

Technical Report Series No. (year)	Expert Committee on Mental Health Report No. or Study Group Reports	Themes
9 (1949)	1	Principles and priorities Education Nurses Fellowships Supply of technical literature to governments Health education of the public Collection of information Advisory and demonstration services to governments Research Alcoholism and drug addiction Maternal and child health Venereal diseases International statistical classification of diseases Morbidity studies Unification of pharmacopoeias
31 (1950)	2	Mental hygiene in public practice Maternity services The infant and the preschool child Separation of the preschool child and the mother Communicable diseases Care of the aged Health education of the public Immigration Health statistics and epidemiologic studies Public health administration Mental hygiene training for the public
42 (1950)	1st Session of the Alcoholism Subcommittee	Alcoholism
48 (1952)	2nd Session of the Alcoholism Subcommittee	Alcoholism
73 (1953)	3	The community mental hospital
75 (1954)	Joint Expert Committee with WHO and UNESCO	Mentally subnormal child

Table 2.1 (continued)

Technical Report Series No. (year)	Expert Committee on Mental Health Report No. or Study Group Reports	Themes
98 (1955)	4	Legislation affecting psychiatric treatment
134 (1957)	5	The psychiatric hospital as a center for preventive work in mental health
151 (1958)	Study Group	Mental health aspects of the peaceful use of atomic energy
171 (1959)	6	Mental health problems of aging and the aged
177 (1959)	7	Social psychiatry and community attitudes
183	Study Group	Mental health problems of automation
185 (1960)	8	Epidemiology of mental disorders
208 (1961)	9	The undergraduate teaching of psychiatry and mental health promotion
223 (1961)	10	Program development in the mental health field
235 (1962)	11	The role of public health officers and general practitioners in mental health care
252 (1963)	12	Training of psychiatrists
275 (1964)	13	Psychosomatic disorders

environmental threats to their development, so that the mental health problems of childhood and youth immediately gained increased notice. One of the committee members, British child psychoanalyst John Bowlby (1907–1990), popularized the view that mental health problems among children were caused by prolonged separation from parents, a concern congruent with the WHO's maternal care project and with the Social Commission of the United Nations, which in 1948 identified the need to study "children who are orphaned or separated from their families for other reasons and need care in foster homes, institutions or other types of group care."[76] Bowlby's theory corresponded with Chisholm's emphasis on the family and other WHO projects related to maternal care. On the basis of the UN Social Commission report, the Mental Health Expert Committee was soon advised to participate in the study of juvenile delinquency and asked to research important medical and psychiatric problems.[77] The initiative echoed other health agenda items that focused on preventing the development of diseases whose future treatment and care costs were likely to be a burden. Expert opinion on juvenile delinquency varied, but many experts supported the UN's program for prevention of crime and treatment of offenders, an agenda developed in tandem with the international mental hygiene movement during the two world wars. Now, however, juvenile delinquency appeared to be a more pressing issue.

For adults, mental health was linked with rapidly changing ways of life after the war. One source of change was technology, especially "automation" and the increasing mechanization of work in postwar society. These concerns were reflected in WHO study group discussions: "Automation … sometimes appears as a savior, sometimes as a devil or menace to the modern world. And both kinds of phantasy, the phantasy of irrational hope, and the phantasy of irrational fear, have created urgent problems in the mental health field."[78] This comment was an opening for psychiatrists to talk about stress among ordinary people, rather than limit their purview to frontline soldiers. Discussion then turned to working conditions in textile factories and coal mines. Experts considered opinions from India, the USSR, and China. The discussion fulfilled, at least to some extent, Hargreaves's appeal to study stressful experiences among ordinary people.

The committee's agenda extended to the peaceful application of atomic energy, perhaps an unusual concern among mental health professionals, but this study group's brief existence marks the WHO's short-lived ideology. In the early 1950s, the fear of radioactive fallout haunted most countries after the USA's nuclear bomb tests at Bikini Atoll in the Pacific Ocean and after a hydrogen bomb test eventually killed a fisherman in Japan.[79] The study group on the mental health aspects of the peaceful use of atomic energy began its activity in 1957, the year the International Atomic Energy Agency (IAEA) was launched in Vienna. In 1953, Dwight Eisenhower, then US president, proposed "the safe use of atomic energy" to the United Nations General Assembly. The formation of the study group, four years later, represented the WHO's early reluctance to respond to and act on crises. Established to protect and enhance health in peacetime, the study group was a subcommittee created by the Executive Board of the WFMH to formulate guidance and advice to the planned IAEA.[80] At a time when atomic energy was seen as extremely important for scientific development, the study group's discussion stands out as a rare instance of a UN agency directly addressing concerns about the risks of scientific progress.

Unfortunately, the views of mental health experts on atomic energy were diverse and vague. Atomic energy was widely considered a threat to health, although this view was refuted by a number of scientists affiliated with the WHO Expert Committee. Before the WHO's effort, this anxiety was reflected in Japanese film director Akira Kurosawa's 1955 film, *I Live in Fear,* which described an aging industrialist's mental breakdown over fears of a nuclear attack. Those members of the discussion panel concerned about the negative effects of atomic energy collected evidence of its neurologic harm. The evidence suggested, for example, that atomic energy might cause brain malformations and alter the brain's electroencephalographic waves. The study group members further argued that atomic energy provoked unhealthy emotional responses, mostly related to fear. The report emerging from this series of discussion was the only comment by the WHO on the effects of such hazards as atomic bomb tests, nuclear waste, and atomic installations.[81] After two years of discussion, the study group quoted British poet Joseph Addison to conclude that its position on atomic energy "ride[s] in the whirlwind, and direct[s] the storm."[82] On May 28, 1959, the WHO signed an agreement with the IAEA, which had previously prevented the WHO from taking a public position, citing its administrative position as an agency of the Security Council rather than the Economic and Social Council, which oversaw the WHO. The agreement marked the closing of the committee's comments, revealing scientists' limited capacity for exercising their judgment within the UN's growing bureaucracy. Not until the mid-1960s would psychiatrists play an effective role in resisting various governments' plan to formalize nuclear power.[83]

All of the projects carried out in the WHO's first decade reflected professional concerns about the devastation of war and its aftereffects on postwar society. Yet despite expert consensus, these projects did not take full advantage of the WHO's efforts to promote cooperation and coordination among national bodies. A bona fide international project had yet to emerge. At the end of the WHO's first decade, G. Ronald Hargreaves wrote that "systematic research" was "only accessible to the long-term study of carefully selected research teams." He added that such teams should be "facilitated by a critical collection of the available evidence" and that data collection should be performed by "one individual who has the benefit of a sufficient amount of technical and clerical help." In Hargreaves's view, not only psychiatrists but also public health workers, psychologists, anthropologists, and other social scientists had made "pertinent observations," and yet they remained uninformed about one another's work. Acknowledging various views and their "critical unification," he maintained that a "single objective investigator" was an "absolute necessity."[84]

The Manageable Project and Four-Man Meetings

In his epidemiological proposal, Hargreaves described a "manageable project" as fulfilling four basic requirements: place, people, money, and method. He understood but did not state explicitly the need to resume the comparative psychiatry initiated by Emil Kraepelin, renowned for his nosological work on mental illnesses, comparing dementia praecox in European and Java patients.[85] Unfortunately, at the time of Kraepelin's death in 1926, his projects remained unfinished. The fundamental difference between Kraepelin's and Hargreaves's ingenuities lay in the fact that the former's work was framed during the heyday of European imperialism, while the latter's work was created against the backdrop of decolonization. Drawing from Kraepelin's work, therefore, Hargreaves envisioned a large project. Hargreaves had trained in Germany, Switzerland, and France; worked as an expert consultant in the Philippines, dealing with the problems of immigrants; and was multilingual. Many of his colleagues at the WHO shared similar cross-cultural and migrant backgrounds. He was thus convinced that the best approach to research would be comparative. From a practical perspective, Hargreaves thought that the project should be conducted from a "centrally situated country, like Switzerland." The WHO's headquarters provided the perfect hub for scholarly exchange and logistics. By the time the flagship research project began to take shape in the WHO, however, this setting was only one of the three critical conditions that had been addressed.

The recruitment of personnel was never easy, and as with most WHO projects, outsourcing facilitated staffing. Hargreaves sought advocates among individuals with similar aspirations and who were more concerned about data obtained from "community studies" than in hospital settings. In 1956, he planned a study group on the epidemiology of psychiatric disorders and proposed a series of meetings that began in September.[86] The gatherings stimulated scholarly exchange among specialists, who were inspired to become the core personnel of the WHO's psychiatric epidemiology project. Paul Lemkau (1909–1992), consultant to the National Institute of Mental Health (NIMH) in the United States, also served as a consultant. Founder of the Division of Mental Hygiene at the School of Hygiene and Public Health at Johns Hopkins University, Lemkau was famous for developing community mental health programs in the United States as a replacement for long-term psychiatric admission.[87] In 1954, he "daydreamed" to Hargreaves that the committee might recruit people from "Norway, Demark, and perhaps in the U.K." for information exchange. In the early 1950s, epidemiological surveys were particularly prominent in Scandinavian countries and Germany. Nordic countries were especially safe to mention or collaborate with regarding their pro-socialist approaches in health care during the Cold War. As for France, Lemkau considered French scholars to be "not good enough" for research of this kind, despite France's long tradition of hospital-based psychiatry.[88]

Beginning in October 1954, during his stint as chief of the Mental Health Section at the WHO, Hargreaves widely circulated an invitation among psychiatrists worldwide who might be interested in the comparative study project and waited for their responses. Thereafter, the correspondence between the WHO headquarters and its potential collaborators snowballed. Hargreaves first solicited advice from Eduardo Krapf (1901–1963), the German-educated Argentinian psychiatrist who later succeeded Hargreaves as chief of the Mental Health Section. Krapf had been a fond supporter of the WHO's plan to compare mental disorders when Hargreaves came to Argentina in 1953 to give his speech "Preliminary Statement on a Research Project Dealing with Mental Health and Disease from a Comparative Point of View," and had forwarded Hargreaves's idea to the NIMH in the US. In response to this proposal, Hargreaves obtained access to several papers written by visionaries such as Carney Landis (1897–1962), a professor of psychology at Columbia University, who pioneered a series of laboratory experiments on human behaviors. In 1938, Landis had published *Modern Society and Mental Disease*, which was essentially an epidemiological survey of mental diseases in America and Europe. In a letter to Hargreaves on April 15, 1953, Landis pondered "the possibility of re-doing [the] book" and emphasized "the changes which have taken place in mental disease statistics since 1935."[89] Hargreaves became deeply intrigued by Landis's research during two months of correspondence, but he voiced his concern about the shortage of funding and suggested that Landis's data, derived from hospital admissions, were strongly dependent on factors other than natural variation in the prevalence of psychiatric disorders.[90] Hargreaves's concern reflected a widespread apprehension among specialists, which could have obstructed the project.

One of the WHO's strengths, however, was the participation of scholars from the Americas. Given this support from other strands of academia (e.g., members of the Pan-America Health Organization), the WHO acquired a privilege not enjoyed by earlier organizations, like the League of Nations Health Organization between the two World Wars or the United Nations Relief and Rehabilitation Administration (UNRRA) during World War II. A number of US psychiatrists expressed interest in Hargreaves's project. However, these scholars differed from the main players in postwar mental health research in the United States, most of whom were linked with the NIMH, believed in biological psychiatry, and were beneficiaries of the pharmaceutical industry. Supporting Hargreaves, for example, was Frederick C. Redlich (1910–2004), at the Yale University School of Medicine, who communicated his interest to researchers conducting projects similar to the WHO's initiative, among them Ernest Gruenberg (1915–1991), Erich Lindemann (1900–1974), and Paul Lemkau, who later became the core personnel in the international field of social psychiatry.[91]

Hargreaves gradually received feedback about the project's feasibility and its potential method. For example, Lemkau, who worked at Johns Hopkins, offered his opinion as a pioneer in preventive psychiatry.[92] While his view echoed that envisaged by experts in Geneva, Lemkau raised the difficulty of traveling to collect data from all over the world and discussed some dubious or inadequate statistical techniques. He was concerned that too few people would be willing to carry out the task but suggested one person in Japan, along with Gruenberg (on the New York Mental Hygiene Commission) and Morton Kramer (1914–1998, United States Public Health Service). Despite Lemkau's doubts, Hargreaves invited him, in 1953, to act on the WHO's behalf and commit to its project in the next year.[93] In fact, despite sharing similar aspirations with other internationalists, Lemkau had earlier, in *Mental Hygiene in Public Health* (1949), been unable to find a satisfactory method for conducting an epidemiology study.[94]

In addition to WHO funding, financial aid came mainly from philanthropic organizations that shared Hargreaves's vision of social medicine. Like the WHO's reliance on the Rockefeller Foundation's indirect contribution, the Mental Health Unit sought help from the Milbank Memorial Fund.[95] Founded in 1905 in New York, the Milbank Memorial Fund had been interested in population studies since its establishment and had played a critical role in scientific research related to human populations in such areas as family planning, fertility, and eugenics.[96] The fund had not, however, encompassed psychiatric science until Hargreaves's invitation. Seeing an opportunity for financial support, Hargreaves wrote to Gruenberg, then director of the fund, suggesting a joint project with the WHO, which he hoped Gruenberg would direct.[97] Gruenberg was a pioneering thinker who shared Hargreaves's perspective on the relationship between social conditions and mental illness. He believed that after World War II, on top of social economic status, anomic conditions and migratory patterns of life could influence mental capacity.[98] Despite his sympathetic stance, Gruenberg did not feel, however, that he could take on the role of handling an international project, noting that the Milbank Memorial Fund had committed itself to a local mental health demonstration project, evaluating selected services. Others who turned the directorship down included Lemkau and Krapf. Nevertheless, Milbank became the main funding body for Hargreaves's project.

While epidemiology was developing a clinical picture and natural history of chronic diseases in the mid-1950s, the WHO's Expert Committee of Health Statistics invited statistical experts to assist different projects.[99] Donald Reid (1914–1977) at the London School of Tropical Hygiene and Medicine (LSTHM) was one of the first medical statisticians who contributed to the mental health project. Together with Bradford Hill (1897–1911), the leading figure in medical statistics at LSTHM, Reid was renowned for his capacity to identify factors causing noncommunicable diseases. While Hill's criteria heavily influenced the search for the cause of lung cancer conducted by the iconic epidemiologist Richard Doll (1912–2005), Reid himself plunged into cardiovascular disease research. Believing that the search for clues about causation had become more systematic, Reid thought that methods of vital statistics could be applied to mental health research. His research indicated that mental status was a variable that influenced the course of cardiovascular and other diseases. For example, mental tension and overwork were among the etiopathogenic factors associated with atherosclerosis.[100] Reid wrote: "the evidence accruing from field observation is circumstantial in that it may be enough to suggest a causal relationship but it cannot give final proof of it."[101] This situation provided the rationale for mental health experts to endorse practical interventions for addressing mental health before the etiology of psychiatric disease had been confirmed.

In addition to Krapf, Gruenberg, and Reid, Swedish psychiatrist Jan Arvid Böök (1915–1995) was asked to join the WHO group because of his expertise in empirical social psychiatry. (At the time, most of the important research in psychiatric epidemiology was conducted in Scandinavian countries.)[102] Krapf, Gruenberg, Reid, and Böök were "temporary advisors," making up the core personnel of the project's study group.[103] Now the dream team formed by the WHO's Mental Health Unit was born, consisting of a capacious administrator, a promising patron, a shrewd statistician, and an experienced practitioner. The "four-man meeting," as it was called, promoted the prominence of their projects. In a letter from Frank Boudreau (1886–1970), president of the Milbank Memorial Fund, to Jerome Peterson, director of the WHO's Public Health Division, Boudreau optimistically wrote of the WHO's bold vision: "[the psychiatric epidemiology project] promises to be as thrilling and probably just as difficult as the pioneering explorations into cholera, typhoid fever, and malaria. If nothing interferes with your plans, all the 'old hands' in public health will envy you and Dr. Krapf, and the excitement of the chase and the WHO itself will grow in the opinion of the profession."[104]

With the recognition of the group of temporary advisors, the Exploratory Meeting on the Epidemiology of Mental Disorders met in Geneva from September 16 to 20, 1957. The four participants had agreed that epidemiology might be a route to understanding the etiology of mental illness.[105] The precise methodology for conducting such a study, however, remained unclear. The four consultants agreed that there was an urgent need to establish "special surveys of baseline incidence rates" for congenital mental abnormalities. They also noted that an "adequate long-term follow-up investigation is needed." Regarding the scale of the project, they felt it was premature to attempt a diffuse "global epidemiology" study, but believed that the WHO could play the role of "intellectual catalyst" to stimulate field workers to travel and meet, and could support the training of specialists in appropriate epidemiological techniques.[106] The meeting also clarified several practical steps, the first being a critical, rather than comprehensive, literature review of epidemiologic studies on mental disorders; as participants noted, "comparisons between the larger or more competent [studies] may be invalidated by differing standards of diagnostic precision."[107] On the basis of this proposal, the attempt to develop standardized classifications and diagnostic criteria for psychiatric diseases gradually intensified.

Practical problems remained. Having formed a well-balanced core group, none of the four experts wanted to direct the long-term project. And research subjects still had to be recruited. Settling on the snowball method of sampling, the WHO Mental Health Unit took another few years to implement the project in a systematic manner.

From Impediment to Collaboration: Ethnographic Approaches

To understand mental disorders at the global level, internationalists in medical research needed to converse and negotiate with anthropologists informed by cultural relativism. While the large-scale international study was taking shape at the WHO headquarters, although its official project name was still lacking, researchers from various geographical regions sent comments to Geneva. Most argued for an ethnological approach and questioned the feasibility of such an ambitious project.[108] Geneva, while the "capital" of international medical studies, was not the only place in the world to be concerned about cross-cultural issues. In 1955, for example, British psychiatrist Eric Wittkower (1899–1983), who had received medical and psychiatric training at the Charité of Berlin and the Tavistock Clinic in London, set up a section of transcultural psychiatric studies with anthropologist Jacob Fried as a joint venture between the departments of psychiatry and anthropology at McGill University in Montreal. One of the most influential individuals to first comment on the tension between culture and mental disorders, Wittkower spent his career looking for possible psychopathogenic dimensions related to culture.[109] In 1957, another influential US psychiatrist trained in anthropology, Marvin Opler (1914–1981), wrote in *Scientific American* that even one psychiatric diagnosis, taking schizophrenia as an example, could actually mean different things in different cultures. However, he did not repudiate the feasibility of comparison. By offering an analysis of schizophrenia in Irish and Italian cultures, he concluded that a social psychiatry approach "could be applied with profit to investigations of other mental disorders beside schizophrenias."[110]

The study section at McGill is still active, mostly renowned for its summer program on social and cultural psychiatry, and its flagship journal, *Transcultural Psychiatry*, is still running today. But a half century ago, Wittkower and Fried's first goal was simply to publish a newsletter and develop a network of psychiatrists to exchange information about the effects of culture on psychiatric disorders.[111] The newsletter editors acknowledged their pride in organizing communication and stimulating cooperation across both continental and national boundaries,[112] and as a result, their efforts appeared to compete with those of the WHO. Immediately after the publication of the newsletter's first issue, therefore, Wittkower sent a copy describing the first survey study to Marcolino Gomes Candau (1911–1983) at the WHO. Wittkower and Fried then circulated a questionnaire among specialists from eighteen countries,[113] and in his report on the responses, Wittkower provided examples of dissimilar manifestations of mental disorders in different countries, followed by further comments on epidemiology. He asserted that "prevalence of mental disorders treated by psychiatrists in various countries varies considerably"; "transcultural comparison of the prevalence of marked disorders is almost impossible"; and "there are differences in the relative frequency of illness, of severity of illness, and of symptomatology and of content in relation to cultural background." Wittkower concluded with the somewhat skeptical comment that "it is obviously impossible to draw any definite conclusions from the heterogeneous material which has arrived from psychiatrists of 18 different countries."[114] He did, however, conclude that "the major psychoses are ubiquitous."[115] Although Wittkower was probably the most critically minded among social psychiatry specialists sharing the WHO's perspective, he noted exceptions among the seemingly impossible comparative studies, some of them in Scandinavian and Asian countries.[116] After the mid-1950s, he and his colleagues spearheaded the discipline of transcultural psychiatry,[117] and today, McGill remains one of the most influential hubs for psychiatrists interested in exchange and debate about the role of culture.

Despite early objections and methodological differences, the WHO was able to proceed with its initiative to compare mental disorders worldwide, charting a middle ground between universal humanity and Boasian cultural relativism as a theoretical basis. Margaret Mead, who served as president of the World Federation for Mental Health (WFMH) between 1956 and 1957, exemplified this middle ground. She was torn between the two extreme approaches but also ardent about the application of anthropology to international relations and public services.[118] Her concept of "one world, many cultures" became one of the bases for neo-Freudian psychiatrists, who rejected the attribution of causation for mental illnesses to the mental capacities of different ethnic groups and instead looked to social and cultural factors determining individual mental integrity. In the meantime, anthropological disciplines, at least in the United States, were gradually weaned from biodeterminism and shifted from studies of "racial types" to "populations."[119] With this momentum, survey studies similar to Hargreaves's initiative became acceptable worldwide.

Also during the early 1950s, UNESCO commissioned the WFMH project Cultural Patterns and Technical Change, led by Mead, to study possible methods of relieving tensions caused by industrialization in various countries. Collaborating with UNESCO, Mead offered anthropological input on international mental health. Unlike the WHO's vertical model, Mead's project aimed to collect and disseminate existing knowledge of various cultures "with respect for their cultural values to ensure the social progress of the people."[120] Sociologists and anthropologists comprised a relatively high proportion of WFMH participants. In 1957, however, a disillusioned Mead left the WFMH, as psychiatric specialists had gradually displaced anthropology's role and cultural contribution. In her words, they "want[ed] to secularize life and [they] want[ed] to destroy all these other systems as wrong and bad and old." .[121] Mead's idealistic objectives were thus left unfulfilled, and the WFMH became less influential.

The end of the 1950s saw nuanced debates over whether social science research design could contribute to comparative studies. In his first newsletter, Wittkower questioned the feasibility of the WHO's planned cross-national study because psychiatrists lacked training in sociology or anthropology and so had only limited assistance from the social sciences.[122] In 1957, while commenting on J. C. Carothers's criticism that modes of simplification for comparisons were needed, Paul Lemkau optimistically expressed to the newsletter that correlations between then-available studies could still be envisaged and a significant generalization would eventually emerge if sufficiently complete, descriptive, and comparative studies were at hand.[123] In September of the same year, twenty-five psychiatrists gathered in Zurich for the Second International Congress of Psychiatry. A roundtable meeting on transcultural psychiatry was convened by Wittkower and Ewen Cameron (1901–1967), both from McGill, revealing diverse attitudes toward the topic. The US delegate, for example, supported the feasibility of transcultural epidemiology as the basis for large-scale studies of mental disorders, while the UK delegate questioned transcultural research, and the Cuban representative favored qualitative studies. Delegates raised the need to standardize terms and profiles of mental disorders and agreed to submit accounts of statistical materials, literature reviews, research facilities, and classification systems to the newsletter. Epidemiology thus became the primary basis for proposed, though still unlikely, comparative studies.

In 1959, Eric Wittkower hired Scottish psychiatrist Henry B. M. Murphy (1915–1987), who joined the McGill group and had a great effect on scientists' attitudes toward international study of mental disorders. Murphy suggested new principles for transcultural psychiatry research: making comparisons, simplification of observed data, contextual determinants, and methodology.[124] More importantly, he viewed cultural traits as behavioral patterns that could be shaped by situational determinants rather than as intrinsic elements of the mind. Murphy had received training in clinical medicine as well as sociology. Before joining McGill's research unit, he had already gained extensive cross-cultural experiences in Malaya and Singapore, where he studied students' mental health and culture-bound syndromes.[125] At McGill, Murphy did not practice as a clinician. He joined the editorship of *Transcultural Psychiatry* as a pure research academic, establishing transcultural psychiatry as a social-scientific discipline. Dialogue thus became possible between transcultural psychiatrists and WHO members, and today Murphy has become an icon of transcultural psychiatry; his *Comparative Psychiatry* is still widely cited as one of the most influential books in the field.[126]

After Hargreaves's proposal for a manageable project, the first large-scale cross-national study by the WHO's Mental Health Unit was not realized until 1965, and was not completely in accordance with its original intention. Participants at headquarters invested the project with their own interests and with an awareness of their own country's niche. Experts involved in the WHO's expanding network agreed, however, that studying mental health issues across cultures was necessary and urgent. As a result, in 1964

Hargreaves's manageable project came to fruition as "The Ten-Year Plan in Psychiatric Epidemiology and Social Psychiatry." It was proposed by the Taiwanese psychiatrist Tsung-yi Lin, who profited from the WHO's outsourcing mechanism. The plan became the prologue for the unit's epidemiological studies of schizophrenia and classification of mental disorders.[127] Most participating scholars agreed that the project was a collaborative effort, not the achievement of any single visionary. Yet it required a bold, charismatic leader, one who was originally a peripheral participant, to reach beyond the realpolitik of postwar science and promote progress toward studying mental disorders.[128]

Birth of an International Team

The study of mental health after World War II saw a conceptual and structural turn. The war affected psychiatric sciences by shifting the concern from soldiers suffering from the war's traumatic effect to the general public. Such a turn emerged not only in the Anglo-American context but worldwide.[129] At that critical juncture, preventive psychiatry was born out of the effort to lessen the burden of war and its aftermath. The focus also shifted from hospital-based treatment of mentally ill patients to the prevention of mental illness in communities. Instead of selecting fit and suitable military personnel to put on battlefields, mental health workers began to concentrate on everyday stresses associated with industrialization and urbanization. To refocus these efforts, the 1948 World Congress on Mental Health became the key event that transformed the practice of mental health care. The congress resulted in a shift from individual and sporadic research to transnational collaboration. The postwar design of the UN's special agencies, in turn, led to the creation of the Mental Health Expert Committee in the WHO and the WFMH. Both reflected Brock Chisholm's vision of "world citizenship."

UN special agencies were designed to fulfill functionalist economists' notions of the spill-over theory, which claimed that improved health would boost economic growth in developing countries, which in turn would "spill over" and promote international cooperation on specific issues. Employed by the new multilateral agency, the WHO's value-free technical assistance scheme and outsourcing strategy also reflected the organization's spirit, which promoted world citizenship. Most concerns raised by the Mental

Health Expert Committee were directly associated with psychiatric professionals' views of postwar conditions, such as the mental health problems of children and young people and the safe use of atomic energy. These issues overlapped considerably with those practitioners in other UN projects were discussing. Mental health professionals formulated these concerns as a collective response to postwar devastation.

The Expert Committee based its cross-cultural project on the consensus that mental health needed to be studied comparatively. It took years, however, for the project to be realized. Apart from the advantageous location of the WHO headquarters in Geneva, problems persisted with personnel, finance, and research methods. In the late 1950s, the first chief of the Mental Health Section, Hargreaves, managed to secure support for the project from the Milbank Memorial Fund, one of the main advocates of population studies in the 1950s. He also recruited four of his colleagues to the leadership group—Eduardo Krapf, Donald Reid, Ernest Gruenberg, and J. A. Böök, who represented different areas of strength in their own disciplines and practices. Techniques borrowed from the fields of public health, epidemiology, and statistics contributed to their methodology, which was challenged by those who favored an ethnographic approach and questioned the project's feasibility. Though impediments slowed the process, they also stimulated reflection that led to a diverse methodology and a project broad in scope. Begun in 1965, the International Social Psychiatry Project thus rested on a foundation of careful preparation.

The transformation of psychiatric disciplines in the early postwar period was a collective response among mental health professionals to the war and its aftermath. Like World War I, the Second World War stimulated interest in psychiatry, and with the effects of environmental stress arousing interest, a new kind of psychiatric science emerged. A disciplinary shift moved psychiatric research and practice away from psychiatric treatment in institutions and toward preventive measures. Recognizing the need to study mental health issues cross-culturally, the new international health organizations facilitated the realization of this professional vision.

Drawing from the idea of world citizenship and functionalist spill-over theories, professionals involved in knowledge making included both an esoteric circle of experts and an exoteric group drawn from outside the WHO. Visionary thinkers carefully planned this new public health approach to mental health research and epidemiology. Their research projects coincided with other projects under development in the UN's special agencies and provided fresh perspectives on mental health issues in different parts of the world. Through complex processes of scientific practice, Chisholm's and Hargreaves's individual views became the foundation of international collaboration. In addition, the decentralized design at the WHO provided peripheral input that became critical to future projects, but the same organizational structure could impede progress, especially when input from the periphery came from those who might not share the WHO's central objectives. The slow incubation of the "manageable project" marks the best example of this *Problematik* in the WHO's Mental Health Unit. The consequent glitches the organization faced as it sought to develop a common language and disease profile in the 1960s will be discussed in the following chapters.

3 Method

On March 1, 1955, an editorial cartoon in the British *Daily Express* commented on the proposal *International Classification of Diseases* made in the WHO (figure 3.1). In the illustration, two chiefs of seemingly underdeveloped tribes discuss the upcoming phase in the classification process, concerning identifying causes of death: "The next course will be two of those UNESCO bods they sent here to find out what witch doctors' patients die of." "UNESCO bods" referred to the personnel sent to investigate diseases among the tribal people in the cartoon. The satirical illustration implied the incomprehensibility of the WHO's project among communities from various cultures and traditions, and indirectly inferred the general population's distrust of the WHO's upcoming project. With the United Nations' plan to standardize disease classifications, doctors would have a common language for communicating with one another. Although the cartoon's message was satirical, its narrative indicated high hopes, a consensus shared by scientists worldwide, or at least in Geneva, where experts were trying to establish methods to achieve their common goal.

Newly established, the WHO was a visionary, idealistic institution. Discussions within the Mental Health Unit's study groups during its first ten years reflected medical scientists' most important concerns. Primarily because of shortages in funding, however, the project Ronald Hargreaves conceived took about a decade to implement. Its slow incubation reveals the difficulty of making even a single team click. Despite the geographical and administrative advantage of its location in Geneva, the WHO faced multiple obstacles, including tensions over definitions, resource scarcity, and cultural barriers.[1] The WHO's objective, however, was to establish useful approaches and practical tools for disease management in developing countries. The

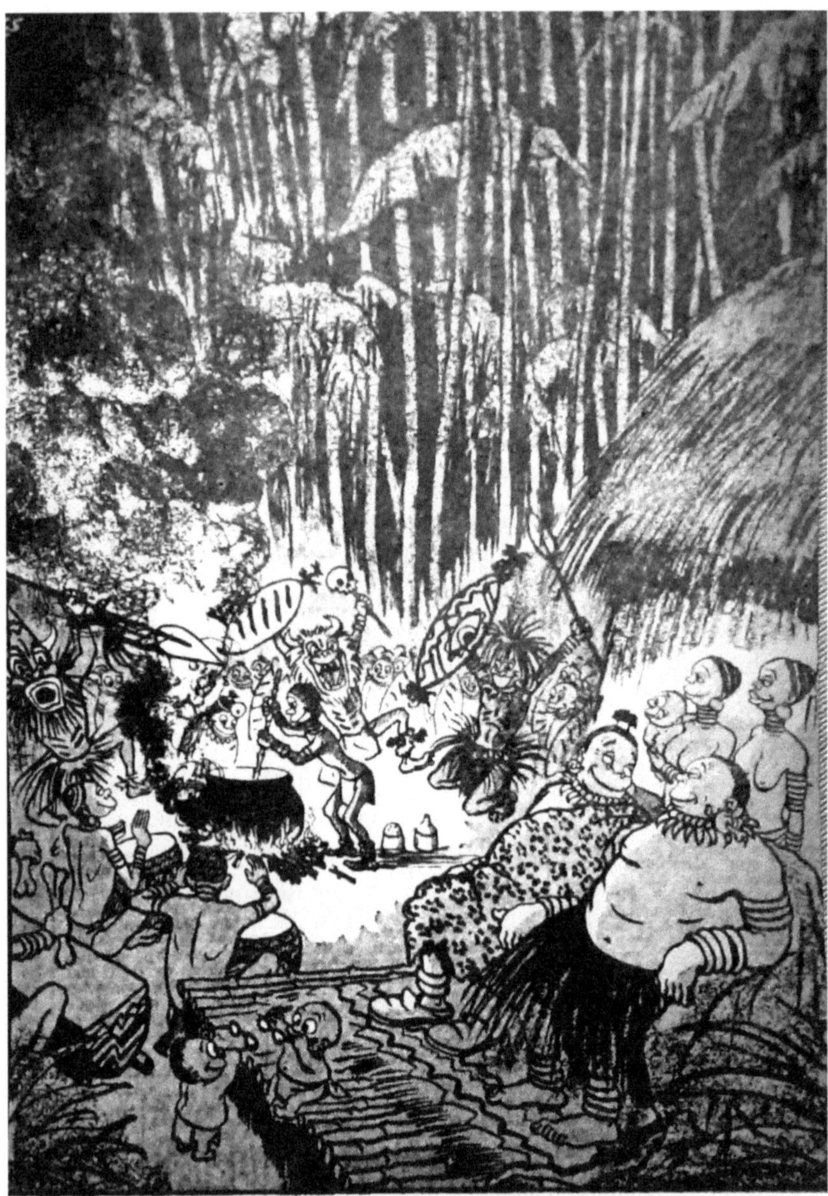

Figure 3.1

"The next course will be two of those UNESCO bods they sent here to find out what witch doctors' patients die of." A satirical comic in *Daily Express*, March 1, 1955. *Credit*: Giles Cartoon, Mirrorpix.

WHO thus had to find a method for studying mental disorders. A robust search for methodology was a precondition for scaling up Hargreaves's "manageable project."

The Need for a Common Language

During the first decade of the Mental Health Unit's existence, experts had already been aware of the urgent need to facilitate its project. In addition to the shared vision among scientists, there was general discontent about existing methods to describe and measure mental disorders. To this end, a standardized classification of mental disorders had to be implemented, and "Development of Standardized Procedures for Case-Finding" formulated a research methodology for international psychiatric epidemiology.[2] Historically, numerous attempts had been made to classify mental illnesses. In the eighteenth century, some systems, like Immanuel Kant's classification,[3] were purely philosophical. Alongside the development of hospital medicine, classifications emerged, some based on symptoms observed among inmates in early nineteenth-century mental institutions. Representative were Philippe Pinel's descriptions of patients in the infamous Salpêtrière in Paris or John Barry Tuke's observations of the Royal Edinburgh Asylum.[4] Comparative studies like Emil Kraepelin's 1919 work on dementia praecox produced other attempts at classification. In fact, by the time the WHO proposed a large-scale, internationally collaborative study on mental health, seven revisions had already been made to the *International Classification of Diseases*, with the chapter on mental disorder having been revised three times under the new structure of an international health organization.

Indeed, starting in the mid-nineteenth century, a few classification systems of mental disorders had been labeled "international."[5] Yet these systems had neither incorporated expertise from the "non-West" nor based their system on any empirical data. Rather, they reflected their writers' idiosyncratic knowledge. By the 1950s, there was a general sense of dissatisfaction with the recently updated seventh revision of the *ICD*. For example, after reviewing the existing twenty-eight different classification systems, the Vienna-born British psychiatrist Erwin Stengel (1902–1973) described the disagreement among psychiatrists over diagnoses and languages used to interpret similar symptoms as "chaotic."[6] Like many other psychiatrists who fled the Anschluss during World War II, Stengel arrived in England in

1938. His critiques have been cited extensively as a precursor of the standardization of mental disorders. Stengel argued that the chaotic individualistic approach in psychiatry would eventually discourage the categorization of mental disorders; the best solution, he wrote, was to conduct a survey and critical examination of the classifications in use.[7]

Nevertheless, experts did not start to see the value of epidemiology as a method for understanding mental disorders from an international perspective until the WHO published its "Eighth Annual Technical Report" during its second decade. In the 1950s, mental disorders were increasingly deemed social and influenced by the effects of external forces on individual mental functioning. In addition to the adverse effect of prolonged institutionalization, social and economic factors were thought to affect individuals' or a population's mental status. Studies were designed and carried out in different parts of the world to test these emerging theories. On a nation-by-nation level, specialists from a range of backgrounds used a variety of methods to study mental illnesses in populations. Many of these specialists eventually became the core personnel that carried out the WHO's projects. They had diverse interests and objectives and fostered their own research within and outside of the WHO. Elements of their collective endeavor also informed the WHO's drive to create an internationally relevant psychiatric epidemiology.

Motivations for developing psychiatric epidemiology differed across countries. The differences were twofold. First was the extent to which psychiatry had been transformed from an instrument for treating and controlling social deviance into a science to prevent the development of mental illnesses. In most countries, psychiatry was no longer employed to control target groups, with the notable exception of a number of European colonies in Africa. The gradual transformation of psychiatric disciplines occurred because psychiatric professionals collectively had called for a response to wartime trauma and the need for rehabilitation. After World War II, American psychiatrists began to believe that the cause of mental illness could be found in the environment. As they started to seek preventive measures, their first step was to conduct mental illness surveys using epidemiology.[8] Among them, Ernest Gruenberg, then working for the Milbank Memorial Fund, believed that a solution for controlling mental illness would emerge from knowledge of the etiology and epidemiology of mental disorders.[9] As psychiatrists used various sampling and grouping techniques in different areas to study the profiles, patterns, and distributions of mental illnesses, their methods also varied.

The second difference in motivations for developing psychiatric epidemiology was the varied perspective on the cause of mental illnesses. As discussed above, psychiatrists in the United States tended to regard mental illnesses as a result of interpersonal relationships and external factors. For example, neo-Freudians gradually shaped clinical practice and factors that were relevant to psychopathology to suit psychoanalysis. Erich Fromm once identified Freud's Oedipal complex as resulting from childhood reactions to parental authority instead of being the instinctive libido that forms the child's character.[10] And neo-Freudian psychiatrist Harry Stack Sullivan also disparaged the importance of instinct and argued that the environment is a more important factor in precipitating individual and social pathology.[11] Coincidentally, the rise of the social sciences corresponded to psychiatrists' search for the causes of mental disorders. In the 1950s, the development of political science, sociology, demography, anthropology, and economics placed their confidence in predicting the outcomes of diseases through controlling social, economic, and cultural variables. In psychiatry, these variables were useful for scientists to search for the root cause of mental disorders.[12] Crucially, during that decade, sociologists at Washington University in St. Louis developed structured interview methods and standardized survey tools to collect large data sets, and instigated a shift from nonspecific surveys of psychiatric diseases to the application of "operational criteria" using statistical validation through sampling, reliability, validity, and other sociological techniques.[13] These methods were central to psychiatric epidemiology in North America and the famous St Louis school of psychiatry. They laid the groundwork for validating the *Diagnostic and Statistical Manual of Mental Disorders* (*DSM*) system.

The WHO's utopian vision inspired medical scientists and public health planners to bring together people from across the globe to work under the same ideological scaffolding. But in the early 1960s, the WHO's global reach was questionable. During its first decade, the United States strategically distanced itself from the United Nations. The WHO encountered difficulty coordinating with the Pan American Sanitary Organization (PASO), and these problems prevented the organization from obtaining financial or technical support from official sectors in North America. The Soviet Union could not effectively collaborate with the organization due to its diplomatic policy. The Arab-Israeli conflict and the controversy over French North Africa also threatened the WHO's visionary ideals.[14] Though experts from different organizations shared likeminded approaches, and though important projects were being initiated, communication between the WHO office in Geneva and PASO began only in the 1960s.

Notwithstanding political interference, the WHO's principle of technical cooperation saw some effective results. Responding to Hargreaves's plan to compare mental disorders worldwide, Eduardo Krapf, who succeeded Hargreaves at the Mental Health Unit, stated in 1953 that such a project should first focus on "the collection of the widely scattered publications on the subject and the provision of a network of correspondents in different professional and geographical areas."[15] Such work, he asserted, should be conducted with the aid of epidemiology. It is worth noting that before the WHO's project, London was already a key center where diverse medical experts with shared visions might collaborate and catalyze a new science. In London were Maudsley Hospital, where practitioners tested new methods to treat war-induced trauma among soldiers and civilians, and the Tavistock Clinic, where they attempted to reconstruct sound minds by exploring human relations. London was also the city where German psychiatrists congregated, after being driven from their homelands by the Nazis.[16] With diverse psychiatrists assembling in the devastated city, London became the home of new theories and methods.

As mentioned in the last chapter, at the end of World War II mental health professionals speculated about possible reasons for the increasing incidence of mental illness, especially neuroses, among soldiers and civilians. During the war, treatment for psychiatric disease among civilians had focused on prevention and favored the civilians' capacity to realize their own allotted wartime duties. Psychiatry also continued to describe the requirements for soldiers on the battlefield (see chapter 2). William Gillespie (1905–2001), who later became an eminent psychoanalyst who promulgated Freud's ideas on sex and death, stated that in the postwar period, "knowledge of what to do, and where to go to do it, coupled with means of reaching the task required of him as soon as possible, is the best preventive of panic and neurosis."[17] Such views on "building a fit man" were common among psychiatrists during the war.

Aubrey Lewis (1900–1975), the first chair of psychiatry at the Institute of Psychiatry (IOP) in London, was one of those who speculated on the issue of war-related trauma. Born in Australia, he trained with Adolf Meyer to become a psychiatrist and moved to London after World War II. Lewis observed that "war brings tribulations and horrors which undoubtedly make people miserable and apprehensive, but the bulk of mental illness in any community is not mainly attributable to recent direct stresses." Lewis was aware of the need to study indirect stressors dissimilar to those experienced on the front line of combat. As he commented, "One cannot speak in the same breath of a community like ours at present and of the people in an occupied and invaded country who have borne over a long period every physical and psychological misery which war can bring."[18] Apart from the burdens war imposed, Lewis foresaw the need to measure the "remediable anxiety and discontents that prevailed during peace."[19]

While prevention remained a component of psychiatry after World War II, the field expanded to study these stressors of peacetime. In a BBC radio talk in 1959, Lewis emphasized,

> mental disorder is not limited to particular countries or particular racial groups. It appears in every society and in every class. It can take rather different forms, according to the culture of the people, and it can be affected by social disturbances, natural catastrophes (such as earthquakes), and by political upheavals: but the basic forms of mental illness appear everywhere.[20]

This claim echoed the appeal made by Hargreaves, who intended to study how "everyday stresses" rather than extreme disaster could cause mental illness (see chapter 2). The WHO's mental health experts were "emphasizing the need for social studies of mental disorder, using methods very similar to those which threw light on the causes and control of epidemics and infectious disease."[21]

Such awareness influenced the work of psychiatrists at IOP. With the development of neuroleptics (today known as antipsychotics) in the early 1950s, severe psychosis suddenly became treatable. The role of hospitals also transformed from custody to treatment. In postwar Britain, surveys investigated the influence of hospital environments on patients' mental functioning, a step reflecting the WHO's call to examine, employ, and improve existing hospital resources. As the number of psychiatric inpatients increased sharply during the first ten years of the WHO's existence, social psychiatrists, such as John Wing (1923–2010) at IOP in London, attested to sociologists' observations of psychiatric hospitals.[22] Wing was director of the Medical Research Council Social Psychiatry Unit at the Institute for twenty-five years.

Claiming that his approach was heavily influenced by Karl Popper's philosophy of science, he developed his thoughts on epidemiology and the nature of classification by focusing on the development of syndromes, by which he also explored the causes of mental disorders.[23] His approach also led him to consider the scientific method as a means to examine mental health hospitals in greater depth, and he led a series of studies that attempted to understand the environment in British psychiatric hospitals.

While Wing's study was ongoing, sociologist Erving Goffman's *Asylums: Essays on the Social Situation of Mental Patients and Other Inmates* (1961) became a bestseller in the English-speaking world.[24] Goffman (1922–1982) conducted his ethnography at St. Elizabeth's Hospital in Washington, DC, and revealed the intimidating everyday life in this "total institution." Goffman's analysis implied that psychiatric administration adversely affected patients' mental health.[25] Wing, however, was not completely convinced by this argument, simply because apart from his criticism of "total institutions," Goffman did not say anything about psychiatric disorders or psychiatric sciences. Wing commented that Goffman "[did] not use conventional psychiatric terminology, and tend[ed] to explain patients' behavior solely in terms of their reactions to the social environment."[26] Wing and his colleagues therefore painstakingly designed a study to examine whether a prolonged hospital stay was associated with adverse effects on schizophrenic patients and to identify the ways such effects could be counteracted or prevented.[27] They collected and compared case studies from three mental health hospitals in England: Mapperley Hospital, Severalls Hospital, and Netherne Hospital. Using standardized interviews and clinical classifications, they rated clinical conditions, ward behaviors, attitudes about discharge, and social conditions. Wing concluded the research report by stating that "[a] substantial proportion of the morbidity shown by long-stay schizophrenic patients in mental hospitals is a product of their environment."[28]

After drawing this conclusion, Wing and his wife, Lorna Wing (1928–2014), expanded the scope of the study. In 1964, the Wings established a project using the Camberwell register, a database for statistical studies, compiled to plan and evaluate local sociomedical services in Camberwell, a South London neighborhood that is part of the Southwark borough. Wing again emphasized the "scientific" purpose of the study. He hoped to collate and translate statistical outcomes into narratives, so that "the most breathtaking scientific discoveries become commonplace." In Camberwell, the

Wings discovered a kind of "social laboratory" and foresaw extending the model elsewhere in the UK, followed by "eventual collaboration with Baltimore [Johns Hopkins], and then the rest of the world."[29] But the Wings' method was time- and energy-intensive. While John Wing established his database of patients, the WHO developed international psychiatric epidemiologic methods for identifying cases and employed Wing's computing method in the later phase of its project.[30]

US National Institute of Mental Health

As principles of military psychiatry were applied to rear-echelon casualties and civilians in noncombat settings,[31] the United States was the other Anglo-American society where survey studies on mental disorders proliferated. Historians have written extensively about the influx of psychiatrists with Freudian psychoanalytic training who had fled from Germany to North America and transformed psychological and psychiatric theory, science, and the broader culture.[32] Another group of US psychiatrists, however, saw the need to expand the scope of prewar and wartime mental hygiene, possibly with the aid of social science. Robert H. Felix (1904–1990), a public health psychiatrist who was originally medical director of the federal Public Health Service, was the first to speak nationally of his vision for the public health services, before the official establishment of the National Institute of Mental Health (NIMH) in 1949. For Felix, the broad principles of public health could be applied to the problem of mental illness much as they had been applied to the problems of tuberculosis, venereal diseases, or malaria.[33] Upon its establishment, the NIMH became the hub that gathered demographic information and trained research fellows in social psychiatry and its related fields.[34]

The NIMH was one of the major research institutions that conducted survey-based epidemiological studies on the increasing burden of care for patients with mental disorders. With its close link with Johns Hopkins University, surveys were conducted in Baltimore as well as in midtown Manhattan before pilot studies proceeded nationwide.[35] These studies, based on interviews and statistics, confirmed a positive relationship between mental health risks and socioeconomic status, as did several surveys later conducted in East Coast cities. The WHO was especially aware of an investigation in New Haven, Connecticut, by Belmont Hollingshead (1907–1980) and Frederick

Carl Redlich (1910–2004).[36] With their disciplinary backgrounds in sociology and psychiatry, respectively, Hollingshead and Redlich investigated the relationship between social class and mental illnesses, and their careful, award-winning epidemiological approach, later known as the Hollingshead Four-Factor Index of Socioeconomic Status, confirmed a strong correlation between poverty and mental illness.[37] In addition, psychiatrists in the West End of Boston, a section of that city slated for demolition, also cooperated with social scientists and city planners to study the influence of urban renewal on mental health.[38] Such work, among others, supported the theories and practices of public health as they applied to mental health in the United States.[39] It was also through correspondence between researchers in the WHO and NIHM that Latin America became the focus of cross-cultural research.[40]

In both the United Kingdom and the United States, studies of different scopes, sampling methods, and sizes of surveyed populations established statistical review as a way of understanding mental disorders. It was the cross-Atlantic diagnostic project on schizophrenia, however, that instigated the cry for a common international language of mental disorders. The dialogue, renowned as the "US/UK diagnostic project," revealed the subjective and unscientific nature of psychiatric diagnoses at the time. The study was led by eminent psychiatrists at NIMH in the US and a team at Maudsley Hospital in the UK (London), where the two teams investigated the reliability of diagnoses of depression and schizophrenia. The study attempted to measure the gap between the two nations in understanding diagnostic and technical terms. The researchers asked American and British psychiatrists to diagnose patients by watching videotaped interviews. The results showed that differences were almost entirely due to diagnostic practices in the two countries rather than differences in the prevalence of mental disorders.[41] Analyzing the same patients, the British psychiatrists diagnosed depression twice as often, while the US psychiatrists diagnosed schizophrenia twice as often.[42] Differences in interpreting symptoms—and thus in diagnoses—implied problems of reliability and differences in psychiatric cultures and strengthened the demand to standardize diagnostic criteria.

The WHO's Scouts and Their International Trips

The experience of US-UK studies on diagnostic differences showed dissimilar approaches to the same mental disorder in the two countries, even within the Anglophone context, let alone among countries of more diverse cultures. In order to solve the problem caused by cultural heterogeneity in scientific research, the first step was for the WHO to consult different "cultural knowledges" before seeking commonality. To this end, the outsourcing design of the organization became critical. To establish a research paradigm on mental health for the Global South, the WHO was keen to include input from non-Western developing countries. Before the establishment of the official Scientific Group, the six regional offices collected preliminary information, and the WHO headquarters then commissioned medical officers hired by the Mental Health Unit to visit countries targeted by the regional offices' recommendation. The medical officers collected useful information for research and identified potential researchers to invite for training or collaboration. For convenience and to save money, meetings between the WHO staff and local researchers sometimes occurred at international conferences. During the harsh days of the Cold War, such trips were planned especially carefully to avoid offending participating states. When the social psychiatry project finally kicked off, the WHO was ready to collaborate with psychiatrists in the USSR, thanks to the death of Stalin.[43] Baltimore native and biostatistician Morton Kramer (1914–1998) reported useful findings after a visit to Moscow in 1963 but suggested that the European regional office of the WHO create a "special sheltered" research fellowship, as requested by the mental health consultant of the regional office to the USSR Ministry of Health.[44] Historians familiar with officially approved scientific discourse have generally assumed that psychiatrists in the USSR were more concerned about biological causes of mental disorders.[45] According to Kramer's report, however, Soviet psychiatrists were aware of the global development of psychiatric theories and mental health research, despite having little contact with Western countries.

The WHO's plans to undertake a study of transcultural psychiatry coincidentally met the aspiration of researchers from developing countries. In 1962, at the Asia Family Conference in the Philippines, where the WHO staff met with local researchers, psychiatrists believed that Asia, with its rich and diverse cultures, had a place in the WHO's plan for international comparison. Agreeing that studying the region required a practical rather than a theoretical or academic approach, conference delegates supposed that small-scale research projects could be done in Asia at relatively low cost and with available personnel. Conference delegates from Asia, however, questioned the contribution of "foreign" experts and challenged the authenticity of their collaboration, claiming that such experts often made "hasty or one-sided observations without proper understanding of the people, language, and culture." Delegates also expressed concerns about communication with those involved in the research and, most important, feared that the WHO's plan applied a Western prototype without proper validation for its use in Asia.[46] These concerns reflected the acrimony evident in debates not only between East and West but also between the Global North and South.

WHO headquarters was aware of research conducted in the Global South, and expert consultants worldwide gradually participated in the organization's plans. Yet a consultant from a distant locale, the island of Taiwan, came to lead the WHO's social psychiatry project. As Tsung-yi Lin, a psychiatrist who spent the war years training in Japan, explained in his memoir, his encounter with Hargreaves occurred because of an article he published with his students in Sullivan's journal *Psychiatry*. "A Study of the Incidence of Mental Disorder in Chinese and Other Cultures" was based on survey research carried out by Lin and his team at National Taiwan University Hospital. One of the first epidemiological attempts in postwar Asia to receive attention from the WHO's Mental Health Unit,[47] the study impressed Hargreaves, who in 1955 took the opportunity to meet Lin during a visit to the WHO's Western Pacific regional office, where they discussed methodology, research outcomes, and the future of Lin's work.[48] Having taken notes of their communication, Hargreaves invited him to serve on an expert committee at the Mental Health Unit of the WHO later that year. Lin then embarked on a worldwide tour.

Despite the imperfections of his research design, Lin's vision for psychiatric epidemiology contributed a blueprint to the WHO's large-scale, cross-national project, initially titled "The Ten-Year Plan in Psychiatric Epidemiology and Social Psychiatry" (referred to here as the International Social Psychiatry Project). It was a collaboration of many disciplines and a realization of the WHO's objective in spirit: the development of a "manageable" international study in which the idea of "world citizenship" was the basis for studying mental illness—universally experienced among all peoples—across national boundaries.[49] The International Social Psychiatry Project also provided the foundation for the globalization of standardized psychiatric diagnoses and research methods in international psychiatric epidemiology.[50] While the WHO considered tentative proposals for its 1960s projects, countries presumed to be suitable for the study—Australia, China, Hong Kong, Japan, and New Zealand—were listed according to priority. A memorandum written by the head of the Western Pacific regional office at the WHO indicated what was sought: a critical review (selective rather than comprehensive) of published articles, either describing new epidemiological methods for investigating mental illness or introducing useful technical modifications of existing procedures to produce a "canon of accepted methods." Hence, the WHO sought the intelligent psychiatrist's guide to epidemiology, and Tsung-yi Lin's research was a well-liked fit with the WHO's criteria.[51]

1961: WFMH and World Mental Health Year

By the end of the 1950s, several centers of mental health research—beyond Geneva and London—shared a tacit agreement that a "new science" should be pursued in response to newly emerging human needs. Thus in 1961, after several years of preparation, World Mental Health Year was inaugurated. Like many similar public relations practices today, the plan successfully attracted attention from governments and funding bodies worldwide. At a conference that year, French psychiatrist Paul Sivadon (1907–1992), a pioneer of cross-cultural psychiatry famous for his work in hospital reform and later at the World Federation of Mental Health, mentioned that psychiatry should "adopt the methods of the ... existing sciences"; he stated that it was "better to understand the mind, which, being intangible, fluid and subtle evaded every scientific approach."[52] To study the mind, Sivadon continued, it was necessary to establish a "common denominator of the motivations, attitudes and behavior of different human groups."[53] Yet he admitted that "the disparity existing between men and cultures will probably prevent [the] values from becoming universal for a long time to come."[54]

To develop the new science, the executive board of the World Federation for Mental Health set up a small committee under the chairmanship of Dutch psychiatrist Henry Rümke (1893–1967), renowned for his effort to characterize schizophrenic gestalt as a key feature for diagnosis. Almost half of the committee's members were anthropologists and social scientists, and its early aim was the collection and dissemination of existing knowledge of various cultures "with respect for their cultural values to ensure the social progress of the people."[55] The committee formulated theoretical principles by clarifying the fundamental concepts of mental health science and eventually came to share a vision and a set of values almost identical to those of the WHO.[56] Later, however, the WHO rather than the WFMH took the lead in the field.[57] As discussed earlier, Margaret Mead, the critical and leading figure at the WFMH, resigned from the federation as its staff of psychiatrists grew and the organization abandoned its original promise of anthropological influence.[58] The study of mental disorders thus became a monolithic discipline led primarily by psychiatrists.

Seeking Peripheral Input

The WHO's International Social Psychiatry Project eventually forged new approaches to the study of social psychiatry across different cultures. Incubation of the project was slow, however. Communications about psychiatric illness and diagnostic criteria remained deadlocked for fifteen years after World War II,[59] despite the establishment of the WHO and the interchange of ideas among member countries. In part, the WHO's work stagnated due to the structure of the United Nations and the way it allocated resources among its specialized agencies. No more than two years passed between drafting the WHO's constitution in 1946 and setting its agenda, but hope for internationalism was soon hampered by the onset of the Cold War, which led to debate about the appropriate role of the United Nations.[60] In addition, the WHO, like other organizations, was constrained by a bureaucracy that hampered its flexibility and slowed decision making. The WHO's growth was further slowed by political strategizing; those who oversaw projects from developed countries wanted to see only small increases in the organization's budgets, even when more money was needed.[61] Money thus became an obstacle to the birth of the International Social Psychiatry Project.

Despite these political and financial challenges, many individuals remained deeply committed to the WHO's overall mission, although the launch of the International Social Psychiatry Project was contingent on multiple factors converging at the right time and place to facilitate collaboration. Geneva was a cosmopolitan city of international influence, where government representatives and professional authorities could meet and become acquainted. Bureaucrats at the WHO stimulated communication among scholars and promoted the interchange of ideas,[62] but the project was nonetheless delayed. One of the most difficult tasks was assembling people from member states to participate.

Only with the formation of the four-man meeting (see chapter 2) did the WHO find a working group that could summon international collaborators. Coming from outside of the organization's bureaucracy, these peripheral participants were bold. Policy makers from less developed countries, including Tsung-yi Lin, wanted greater representation in leadership. While the WHO was developing an early mental health project, Education and Mental Health, Lin wrote to the director-general: "our colleagues in Asia have been making continuous [efforts] to convene a meeting of this kind in [Asia]" because "they played an important role in the selection of the theme." Lin also felt that the Western Pacific regional office's "encouraging willingness to send two representatives [in 1958] is a reflection of this enthusiasm." He added, "I realize that the relationship of non-governmental organizations with the WHO is with Headquarters, but, for the sake of the future effect of this meeting on the promotion of mental health in [Asia], I wonder whether this matter could be re-considered and WPRO permitted to send at least one representative financed from regional funds?"[63] As the WHO headquarters

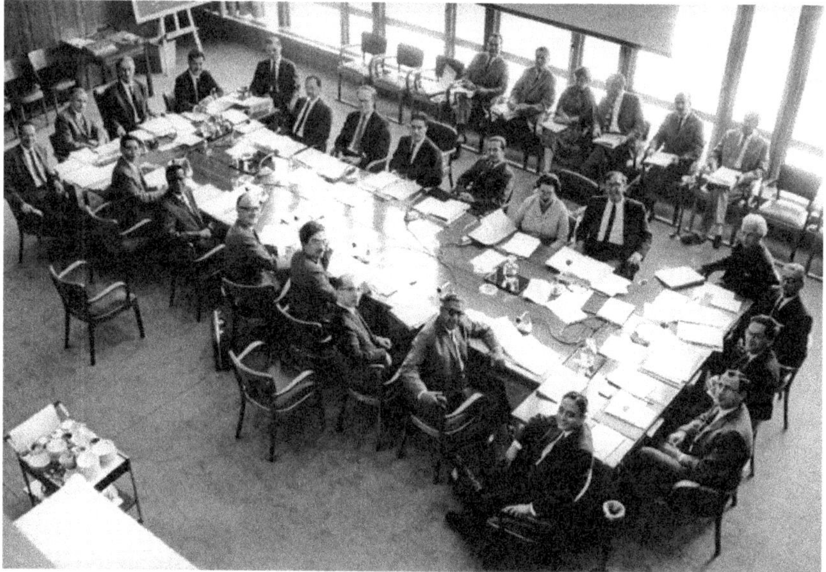

Figure 3.2
The WHO Mental Health Section Seminars, with Tsung-yi Lin sitting in the upper-left corner.
Source: Eileen Brooke Papers AIMG-0799, box 1.
Credit: Bianco Studio

lacked sufficient resources, the voices from regional offices were relatively well received. Lin then assumed an important position in Geneva.

The International Social Psychiatry Project was technically an "intragovernmental" endeavor, but its realization required "non-state" participants. The WHO's advisory services played a central role in facilitating technical cooperation, in contrast with the sluggishness of financial aid and operational activities.[64] Recruits from the advisory services, recommended by the regional offices based on the professional contributions they had achieved in their own countries, were essential to a number of the WHO's thematic projects. They often professed views different from those of their respective nations, however, and to some degree spoke from personal perspectives rather than their official positions as national representatives. At the WHO, many of these recruits also offered expertise that differed substantially from the mainstream theory and practice in their countries of origin. For example, Eduardo Krapf, who came from Argentina, did not represent the psychoanalytic culture there. Similarly, American epidemiologists based at NIMH were affiliated with neither mainstream psychoanalysis nor biologically based theories.[65] Scientists from Asia faced their own dilemmas in a postcolonial world: whether to participate as representatives of their nation states or as internationalists who fully embraced the WHO's vision.

Language was still a pressing issue. Although participants shared experiences and visions, they needed a standardized set of definitions and terms to communicate. The lack of standardization was first recognized as a problem in the early 1960s, when the organization's main work on world mental health and the development of the cross-national collaborative project were preceded by a survey and a series of seminars. The aforementioned UK-US conflict regarding the diagnostic approaches between psychiatrists in two countries marked one of the most significant examples. In 1960, seeking to establish priorities for mental health projects, the WHO conducted a survey of resources and facilities available for future international projects.[66] At the Fifteenth World Health Assembly, in 1962, technical discussions were devoted to mental health projects in public health planning.[67] Technical cooperation within the WHO was typically stimulated by the advisory services, whose members were usually outside of Geneva. During the first half of the 1960s, a number of seminars addressed the integration of mental health into the public health services in countries such as Mexico (1962), Argentina (1963), the United Kingdom (1964), and Jamaica (1965).[68] While conducting these seminars, however, the WHO's experts were aware that lack of standardization was a central concern. For example, Eileen Brooke (1926–1989), the British statistician hired by the Mental Health Unit, commented in her review of Lin's ten-year project that "[the] increasing number of reports in the last few decades have provided much-needed information. However, the reported results of various studies are not comparable because of different methods of investigation employed; some of the results were drawn from hospital studies, some from field surveys, others from lesser known professions." In the early 1960s, without a systematic, standardized method of reporting results, studies were deemed "premature," lacking "universal significance in the etiology of mental disorders."[69] As experts agreed, understanding psychiatric morbidity required consistent definitions and reporting procedures for mental disorders worldwide.

To counter methodological shortcomings, Lin and WHO colleague C. C. Standley wrote "The Scope of Epidemiology in Psychiatry," which became the key document for the WHO to establish the canon of psychiatric epidemiology, thus facilitating international collaborative research.[70] They presented the paper at the Conference on Techniques of Epidemiological Surveys of Mental Disorders, held in the Western Pacific regional office in Manila in 1962. Underscoring the treatability of mental disorders, Lin and Standley reemphasized that mental disorders are diseases that fit the epidemiological definition of morbidity. Surveying a comprehensive forty-year review of prevalence rates, they stressed the need to formulate statistical measures for psychiatric epidemiology. The Lin-Standley report stood out for its emphasis on underdeveloped countries as laboratories for understanding the universality of mental disorders against the backdrop of postwar rehabilitation and development. In their discussion of the Asian experience, Lin and Standley "[did] not pretend to be comprehensive, but point[ed] out that some of the research done in Asia [had] already proved its scientific quality and practical, operational value."[71] The conference thus laid the foundations for psychiatric epidemiological studies in other countries, and the WHO's Mental Health Unit looked for experts outside Geneva with experience in "cohort studies of mental disorders" and "cross-cultural research."[72]

No single person was the mastermind of the International Social Psychiatry Project. Rather, project scientists shared a worldview and an image of a new scientific canon. The exchange of ideas among the WHO, the London Group (such as John Wing, Aubrey Lewis, and their connections), the NIMH, and other peripheral groups and individuals was central to this epoch-making project. During the late 1950s, Wing's population-based study of the admission and readmission rates of psychiatric patients, conducted with other psychiatrists in London, foreshadowed these researchers' Camberwell register and the launch of the Social Psychiatry Unit Medical Research Council in 1964. By then, the epidemiological information system and the sampling frame of the London Group had been established.[73] Meanwhile, in 1963, NIMH had received a generous grant of $500,000 from the United States Public Health Service to establish the National Clearinghouse for Mental Health Information.[74] These research centers became the launch partners of the WHO Mental Health Unit.

Efforts to expand the scale and scope of epidemiological psychiatric studies were similarly decentralized. In the autumn of 1962, Lin, then an expert consultant, visited NIMH in Bethesda, Maryland, and learned of an ongoing study there, which encouraged him to conduct a larger one.[75] Then, during the seventeenth annual meeting of the WFMH in Bern in August 1964, discussion groups considered several topics for the WHO's mental health projects, including transcultural epidemiology and documentation of mental health data. Joy Moser (1921–2001), the veteran assistant at the WHO Mental Health Unit who joined the organization in 1950 and was later known for her work on alcoholism,[76] closely collaborated with Morton Kramer of the NIMH on the initial preparation of an international guide to the collection of psychiatric statistics. She was the WHO representative who had visited several regional offices in the early 1960s to review the collection and analysis of information on psychiatric resources. Earlier in the year, Moser had also represented the WHO at the WFMH conference of Information Centre Correspondents in March and had held further discussions on collaboration between the WHO and the NIMH with the new chief of the NIMH Clearinghouse for Mental Health Information.[77] With this background, discussion at the WFMH Annual Meeting focused on setting up case registries, which were deemed crucial for mental health research.[78]

In April 1964, the WHO announced objectives for its psychiatric research unit. Its Scientific Group on Mental Health Research stated that it

> was acutely aware of the very wide scope of the subjects which are included under the general topic of Mental Health Research. In selecting some areas and some topics within these areas, as being particularly suitable for research activities on the part of the WHO, the Scientific Group wished to emphasize that it would be necessary to seek the advice of small groups of experts in these several fields in order to work out the precise details of the research undertakings which they have indicated.[79]

The group's initial aspirations were large, directed mainly toward two areas—social psychiatry informed by psychiatric epidemiology and biological psychiatry, which was still deemed important. Nevertheless, although the WHO team included specialists in genetic studies, the core staff of the Mental Health Unit was largely composed of social psychiatrists. Epidemiology became its core focus.

As the establishment of a common terminology became central to plans for cross-national mental health studies, the WHO's International Social Psychiatry Project began its work devoted to comparative research. In 1965, a sum of $25,000 (approximately $202,000 in 2021 dollars) was committed to establish three scientific groups: the first would address nomenclature, classification, and statistics; the second, epidemiological methodology; and the third, genetic problems. The first group secured the greatest funding, at $13,000.[80] These three projects (particularly the first two) echoed the priorities identified by researchers in London and Bethesda and at the WFMH, which had just relocated to Geneva.[81] How, then, did the WHO determine the course of international collaborative research? When organizing a seminar, the WHO headquarters would select a group of twelve international experts plus representatives of a local group from the host country and representatives from neighboring countries.[82] Documents prepared by the Mental Health Unit described activities in the field research centers (FRCs) as "national" rather than "country" activities,[83] terminology intended to reassure this nationalism of postwar nation states. The medical officer of the project was authorized to travel extensively, to conduct roundtable meetings organized by regional offices, to raise funds,[84] and to look for prospective advisors.[85] In addition, particularly for the International Social Psychiatry Project, investigators were required to travel to all FRCs to familiarize themselves with the language environment, research settings, and cultural contexts.

Realization of the "Common Language" Project

The International Social Psychiatry Project that Tsung-yi Lin proposed to the director general of the WHO was arguably a "hit and run" plan, which, as in baseball, involved moving forward without knowing in which direction the ball (or project) would go. The strategy was designed to take advantage of momentum, with some work starting immediately, even though "there was not yet available a well-defined research technique for such a study."[86] The

International Social Psychiatry Project included four subprojects—or perhaps more accurately, four mutually complementary projects—in an overlapping sequence:[87] (1) standardization of international classification of psychiatric diagnoses, (2) comparative research on specific mental disorders, (3) research on mental disorders in geographically defined populations, and (4) training in epidemiological techniques. The first two subprojects began immediately, with their results intended to inform the latter two. Simply from the first two items, we know that experts were already trying to classify mental disorders before their universal profiles had been confirmed.

Preparation for the ninth edition of the *International Classification of Diseases* (*ICD-9*) spurred these subprojects. In 1965, efforts to produce and disseminate international standards for psychiatric diagnosis, classification, and statistics addressed Stengel's earlier critique that the system of disease classification was chaotic, and that there should be a new initiative to "investigate present trends in psychiatric classification used for clinical, statistical and research purposes."[88] The first project, which started in London in October 1965, consisted of eight yearly seminars, beginning with discussion of "problems related to classification of mental disorders, diagnostic variation, and national projects of psychiatric statistics." The meetings were attended by a core group of twelve experts from different schools of psychiatry, augmented by local experts at each hosting center. The seminars initially included only a small circle, primarily experts from the London Group and mainly Maudsley psychiatrists and their long-term collaborators.[89] This group eventually expanded by disseminating information to individuals willing to collaborate, and ultimately included experts from more than forty countries.

The seminars originally were held in both developed and developing countries—among them Chile, France, Israel, Japan, Norway, Poland, the UK, the US, and the USSR[90]—reflecting diverse geographic locations, cultures, and political ideologies. In the longer term, however, difficulty organizing international travel led to the replacement of Chile, Poland, and Israel with more accessible countries. The yearly seminars were held in the cities shown in figure 3.3.[91] Five of the seven were in Europe, and none was in the southern hemisphere.

From the start of the classification subproject, professionals were aware of other needs, such as the need for methods to assess disabilities associated with mental disorders and psychiatric classifications for use in primary

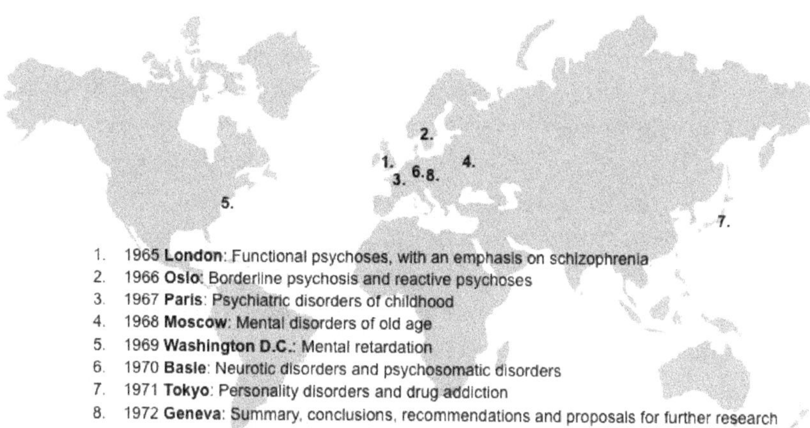

Figure 3.3
Countries hosting the WHO mental health seminars.

care.[92] They also assumed that any classification system used for treatment could be changed over time. At the beginning of the project, the WHO identified and recruited experts according to their scholarly qualifications, their familiarity with statistical science, their familiarity with professionals in the headquarters, and their long-term commitment to the project.[93] The core group also pinpointed functional psychoses, especially schizophrenia, as the most important diseases for study, as members agreed that schizophrenia had well-recognized symptoms worldwide. Nonetheless, the WHO's plan encompassed all major disease categories, ordered according to priority.[94]

The second subproject attempted to attest the universality of mental disorders. Initially titled "Comparative Research on Specific Mental Disorders," it was meant to test and apply diagnostic concepts developed in the disease classification project by examining the profiles of specified mental disorders. The WHO first had to develop complementary uses of standardized methods for rating symptoms. In 1966, after one year of planning, the second subproject launched the renowned International Pilot Study of Schizophrenia (IPSS). Practical concerns had again led experts to choose schizophrenia as their focus, commenting in their meeting that "Confusion and disagreement that still exist over diagnoses, [the] natural history of the illness and the response to the various treatments for schizophrenia make an international study desirable."[95] Substantial work had already addressed the epidemiology of schizophrenia, and yet it was more than the "universality" and "seriousness of its effects" that led to the choice of this disease.[96] Experts had earlier agreed that "a working definition of schizophrenia can be evolved during the London meeting in 1965 and used in the comparative studies,"[97] and stated that "agreement on a definition of manic-depressive psychosis can be relatively easily reached,"[98] indicating a hope to expand the study to include other psychiatric diseases.

The objectives of the IPSS were ambitious but practical. By identifying cases of schizophrenia in a selected set of countries with contrasting sociocultural situations, the researchers aimed to develop uniform instruments to diagnose the condition, to assist in training personnel for collaborative research, and to develop an organizational framework for ongoing research on other mental disorders. John Wing of the Institute of Psychiatry in London suggested that the location of the study should be an area convenient for research, with a homogeneous population and little population movement—that is, "racial homogeneity" with low rates of in- and out-migration. It should have strong psychiatric leadership, a good existing network of services for a population of about one million, and available demographic and sociological data. Most important, the study had to include developing countries.[99] Experts proposed a study that included six areas, with one in the USSR and at least one in Asia. In the first round of selections, twenty countries (both developed and developing) were identified as potential sites.[100] By the beginning of 1966, the list had been reduced to eight: Aarhus, Denmark; Agra, India; Cali, Colombia; Ibadan, Nigeria; London, UK; Moscow, USSR; Taipei, Taiwan (then China); and Washington, DC. A year later, Prague, then in Czechoslovakia, was added.[101]

From September 27 to October 1, 1965, the technical meeting on comparative research was held in Geneva with participants from France, Scandinavia, Colombia, the UK, the US, and the USSR. At the meeting, psychiatrists, sociologists, and psychiatric geneticists discussed possible methods of case-finding, measurement of psychiatric impairments, measurement of factors affecting the evolution and duration of illness, and sociocultural factors that influence disease outcome.[102] The group planned annual meetings at which principal investigators could collaborate with an ever-widening pool of researchers, with their work reviewed every three to five years.[103]

At the initial meeting, Wing proposed a method to standardize the diagnosis of schizophrenia, in which each clinical interview would be recorded as a twenty-minute film, to be used to establish a standardized symptom-sign inventory and questionnaire. Investigators reached an agreement on interview instruments, which were then translated into different languages. Although experts pursued "objective and reliable ratings" in measuring the impairment of schizophrenic patients and the sociocultural factors affecting disease outcomes,[104] achieving agreement on quantitative ratings rather than qualitative descriptions required enormous effort.[105] While the IPSS was identifying centers and principal collaborators, the US/UK project was preparing its first comparative study of hospital admissions in London and New York. Both the IPSS and the US/UK diagnostic project ultimately employed a structured interview method, which became the Present State Examination (PSE).[106]

The IPSS was carried out in three stages: preliminary, initial evaluation, and follow-up. During the preliminary phase, the principal investigators (mostly those who had developed the PSE interview instrument in London and Geneva) organized their FRC teams, trained their interviewers, and tested procedures by selecting and assessing twenty-six patients. In the initial assessment phase, a total of 1,202 patients from nine FRCs were analyzed and then diagnosed: 811 patients were diagnosed with schizophrenia; 164 with affective psychosis; and 227 with other psychoses or nonpsychotic conditions. Patients were then selected for the IPSS by diagnosis. Eligible patients had to be between fifteen and forty-four years old and have had psychotic symptoms such as delusions, hallucinations, or other strange and inexplicable behavior not associated with mental retardation. Having selected their patients, investigators administered the PSE, followed by other instruments including the Psychiatric History Schedule and Sociodemographic Schedule.

The IPSS was the first large collaborative study to confront the problem of translating conventionally accepted symptoms common to European psychiatry into non-European languages. The study was not easy at all, as the translation labored to achieve the intended comprehensiveness while remaining aware of possible incommensurabilities among different languages. For the IPSS, the PSE was translated into seven languages by developing a system of translation and reiterative back-translation, which depended on finding equivalence of meaning rather than translating literally, word by word. The IPSS required subsequent studies for validation, but it confirmed the feasibility of international collaboration. It also convinced researchers that schizophrenia had a global profile of symptoms. Nevertheless, the results also suggested that symptomatically similar patients may differ greatly in course and outcome and that the illness "appears to be less severe in the developing centers."[107] This unexpected outcome stimulated the WHO to conduct yet another study while entering the next phase of international collaboration.[108]

The subsequent study, the Determinants of Outcome of Severe Mental Disorders (DOSMED), was the first mature attempt to conduct psychiatric epidemiological research at the international level. The sampling and statistical techniques were more carefully designed, and the number of FRCs was increased. Taipei was also removed from the study. The complete list of study areas for both the IPSS and DOSMED appears in table 3.1.[109] Through DOSMED, researchers located, for the first time, the psychopathology's common ground internationally, through data showing a similar incidence of schizophrenia across areas. The success of the study encouraged epidemiologists to design more international studies in psychiatric epidemiology

Table 3.1
WHO Field Research Centers (FRCs) collaborating in the International Pilot Study of Schizophrenia (IPSS) and the Study of Determinants of Outcome of Severe Mental Disorders (DOSMED)

Country	IPSS	DOSMED
Colombia	Cali	Cali
Czechoslovakia	Prague	Prague
Denmark	Aarhus	Aarhus
India	Agra	Agra
		Chandigarh
Ireland		Dublin
Japan		Nagasaki
Nigeria	Ibadan	Ibadan
Taiwan	Taipei	
UK	London	Nottingham
USA	Rochester	Honolulu
		Washington, DC
USSR	Moscow	Moscow

focusing on nonpsychotic diseases (e.g., depression).[110] Other follow-up studies on schizophrenia continued at individual FRCs.[111]

Tsung-yi Lin's earnest plan failed to be completed on time. Like most multisite scientific research, coordination kept pushing back the progress. In the meantime, Lin was also planning to relocate to North America. Before he left the WHO, only the first two subprojects had progressed according to schedule. After Lin relocated to Michigan in 1969, Norman Sartorius (1935–) took the helm, continuing with the subprojects on mental disorders in geographically defined populations and the training in epidemiological techniques, as well as other projects derived from the completed subprojects. While these programs were conducted, many research instruments (including questionnaires and technology for data analysis) advanced. The WHO's first two subprojects, however, had great historical significance for the development of modern psychiatry. The first, seeking international standardization, created a common language for psychiatrists; the second, the comparative research on specific mental disorders, provided scientific evidence for epidemiological assumptions about the universality of psychopathology.

Significance of the WHO's International Social Psychiatry Project

Like most projects under the aegis of the United Nations, the WHO's International Social Psychiatry Project was influenced by the geopolitical situation of its era. By the time the project was launched, the WHO was greatly influenced by international relations despite its focus on the apolitical "world." The unrest in Israel and Chile prevented these countries from serving as FRCs even though they had been in the original proposal. The WHO successfully joined with the Pan American Health Organization (PAHO), but in the shadow of McCarthyism in the US, the project could not exempt itself from concerns about communism. After project participants were informed that delegates from the USSR would be included in their work, tensions ran high. For example, G. C. Tooth from the Ministry of Health in London asked that his communications with Geneva be kept confidential and his part in the project be kept quiet.[112] In 1965, experts from the USSR were invited to arrive in London four days ahead of the first classification meeting, "for the purpose of becoming more oriented to 'Western' psychiatry before the discussions begin, and to inform [the participants] of present practice in the USSR,"[113] even though Soviet psychiatrists were aware of the development of modern psychiatry in the so-called Western bloc. When the group met, Tooth distanced himself from any informal gathering with the "crowd," which included the four Russian representatives.[114]

Against the backdrop of the Cold War, the WHO sought to balance worldwide contributions of expertise and did not welcome the participation of the USSR's politically allied countries. In 1968, before the fourth classification seminar in Moscow, Marcolino Gomes Candau, director-general of the WHO from 1953 to 1973, expressed his hope that those in the USSR "responsible for arranging [the] seminar would accept without any deletions the list of the participants originally discussed with the Mental Health Unit staff."[115] In turn, the USSR delegates expressed their wish that the seminar include delegates from East Germany.[116] The USSR Ministry of Health and the WHO then agreed that the WHO would not cover travel expenditures for Soviet participants.[117]

The spirit of internationalism that had prevailed in the early postwar period—between 1946, when the WHO's constitution was signed in San Francisco, and 1948, when the WHO was established in Geneva—had ebbed. The UN was granted the authority to regulate the WHO's membership. In the following year, controversies among member states relating to issues other than medicine led to the withdrawal of several Eastern European countries, and after 1950 other disputes involved North Korea, East Germany, North Vietnam, and the representation of China.[118] In the Mental Health Unit's International Social Psychiatry Projects, Taiwan became an FRC not only because the country was project director Tsung-yi Lin's motherland but also because it had powerful supporters in its claim to represent China, even though China had been identified as a country requiring special attention for mental health development. For Lin's successor, Norman Sartorius, however, the idea that Taiwan could represent all of China was unrealistic.

When Lin left in 1969, four years after the International Social Psychiatry Project had commenced, the Mental Health Unit had completed half of its stage-based tasks. For the common language project, five seminars had been conducted. The research method for the IPSS had also been fully established. Subsequent researchers could continue according to the norms established in the project's preliminary stages. When Taiwan left the WHO in 1971, the NIMH funded follow-up studies. After leaving the Mental Health Unit, Lin moved to Michigan but eventually took up permanent residence in Vancouver. While teaching at the University of British Columbia, he also assumed the presidency of the World Federation for Mental Health, where he replicated his experience at the WHO by recruiting psychiatrists worldwide.

The WHO model thus began to play a significant role in the development of mental health research. Many elements of the International Social Psychiatry Project—the WHO's position as a political entity, the relationships it fostered, and the accumulation of daily detail that generate the culture of an organization—defied easy categorization but collectively influenced its success. In the following chapter, I will discuss in greater details the relationship between the WHO and its member states by looking at the activities of experts, on which the project heavily relied.

4 Experts

In this and the next chapter, I would like to rewind the timeline a little to address two important factors concurrently shaping the WHO's operation. At a symposium organized by the London-based Ciba Foundation in Montreal, on February 23, 1965, scientists researching transcultural psychiatry discussed schizophrenia in different cultures. The International Social Psychiatry Project had just recently begun, and Sir Aubrey Lewis opened the event. Psychiatrists, anthropologists, and scientists from different countries promoted international cooperation in medical and chemical research. Opening the symposium, the head of McGill's transcultural psychiatry research unit, Eric Wittkower, asked panel discussants about the gap between standard nomenclature and indigenous etiological theory on schizophrenia. Henry B. M. Murphy replied reservedly to Wittkower that he did not think the Canadian survey contributed to a current understanding of the gap. Murphy continued: "Much more needs to be done in this area. The word 'schizophrenia' is used for a host of conditions which eventually, perhaps, we will be able to separate out. The tendency at the moment is to use the word as a blanket term to cover many syndromes."[1] Tsung-yi Lin, then medical officer of the WHO's Mental Health Unit, supported Murphy's call for more rigorous research, but he also sought to downplay the cultural disparity of schizophrenia, saying: "I do not think the cultural variation is as great as one might have presumed. It seems to me that the education and training background of the psychiatrist is more decisive than cultural variations in the identification of symptom-complexes."[2]

The two experts exemplify the dissimilar perspectives of what expertise meant to the key players in the field of international psychiatric research. For those who came from the "West," feasible research had to be developed to understand things yet to be explored. Survey studies were never enough. For those who came from the "non-West," training in modern psychiatry was their primary concern.[3] And that is exactly why the fourth item in Lin's proposed Ten-Year Plan in Psychiatric Epidemiology and Social Psychiatry focused on the education of psychiatric professionals in developing countries (see chapter 3). These two dichotomized perspectives shaped the space of international collaboration on mental health research. Different kinds of experts were involved in the WHO's flagship International Social Psychiatry Project, and their activities at home and internationally determined the project's shape. Originally, the WHO hoped to summon talented individuals to represent their own cultures and contribute to idealistic projects in the co-production of knowledge. It was, however, their homogeneous training background that mattered.

During the first two decades of the WHO's Mental Health Unit, the painstaking process of forming its "manageable project" reflected not only its institutional ecology and modus operandi but also the long negotiation among scientists regarding knowledge production. The WHO's organizational advantage helped the unit to accelerate the process, and its agency of experts mobilized the process of transnational knowledge making. This chapter will look at how these experts from diverse backgrounds reached an agreement. If consensus was limited, what did the product of the process represent? In what space did the WHO and member states exchange knowledge, share methods, and collaborate to carry out research? In effect, the WHO's "decentralized" modus operandi and the dreamscapes of international local experts jointly created a space for collaboration. In the dreamscape, experts could exercise their aspirations as a form of "sociotechnical imageries" that were "collectively held, institutionally standardized, and publicly performed visions of desirable futures."[4] In such a space, only limited knowledge exchange occurred. More important, it was a space in which visionary scientists who had similar backgrounds and who shared a similar image of the universality of mental disorders could bond with one another.

To recap the story in the previous three chapters: by the 1950s, an emerging, cross-national psychiatric discourse sought to compare the symptoms of mental illnesses on the basis of universal psychopathology and a shared international system for classifying disease. Psychiatric epidemiology, from the local to global scale, supported this idealistic effort. The WHO thus embarked on an empirical project and, before the rise of global developmentalism, applied a vision of health as a human right for all "world citizens." As the WHO's scientists debated the causation and classification of mental disorders, psychiatric epidemiology became an important method for verifying diagnostic criteria and identifying disease patterns and trends. At the WHO, Brock Chisholm's concept of world citizenship became the theoretical foundation for a "manageable project" in social psychiatry that would apply epidemiology to study mental disorders.

Consistent with the concept of "world citizenship," the WHO claimed to establish common diagnostic criteria and universal epidemiological profiles of mental illnesses that varied minimally across countries, ethnicities, and cultures.[5] Before World War II, psychiatry developed in the "non-West," predominantly in different colonies, had conformed to notions of racial science, supported by the technology of the time. Because racial science supported colonial governance, the discipline of ethnopsychiatry first emerged to construct colonial subjects. Psychiatric theories and practices thus demonstrated colonizers' intellectual superiority and legitimized government control over colonial subjects, who were deemed mentally inferior. Categories and pathologies of mental illnesses were created that demonstrated the colonial subjects' substandard mental capacity and maladaptation to modern life. Psychiatric custody separated European patients from the colonized "native insane," and psychiatric institutions served as instruments of colonial control.[6] In contrast, during the worldwide process of decolonization, the pursuit of universal diagnostic criteria and metrics based on surveys of mental disorders represented a paradigm shift through which psychiatry could be transformed from an imperialist instrument to a worldwide system of treatment and care.

Despite internationalists' efforts to transform the discipline to support global emancipation, psychiatry still reflected a colonial past. Setting aside the stagnated formation of the African regional office, case studies documenting postwar practice in postcolonial societies, for example, reveal the influence of psychiatric rhetoric on epidemics of mental disorders. Variation also suggested a need for cultural autonomy amid the discourses of postwar state building.[7] Under the structure of the United Nations and its specialized agencies, the psychiatry developed from Geneva was driven by clinicians and scientists seeking to shape postwar global society along universal and democratic principles. The discipline they promoted was thus a departure from prewar Eurocentrism. Calling for international collaboration, they sought experts from non-Western locales and drew from research conducted in developing countries. Beginning in the mid-1950s, non-Western survey studies exerted a significant effect on the WHO's International Social Psychiatry Project and on the revision of the ICD system. Developing countries contributed both personnel and methodology to large-scale international epidemiological research shaped by the WHO's scientific ideology.

To best characterize the relationship between the WHO and developing countries, perspectives from the Third World—Asia, Africa, and Latin America—which came late to modern medicine, are especially illustrative. Did such relationships corroborate Javed Siddiqi's early criticism that the collaboration was a vertical and top-down approach despite the horizontal design of the organization?[8] Were these regions working with the WHO through a "marriage of convenience," as historian of global health Anne-Emanuelle Birn describes the decades-long partnership between the Rockefeller Foundation and the Mexican government in the 1920s?[9] Or was the relationship with the WHO like the "trading zone" described by Peter Galison, in which scientists from different paradigms and disciplines collaborate for dissimilar purposes, yet yielding the same outcome?[10] Ideally, the WHO's structure should have enabled international teamwork with contributions in equal measure. But in reality, formal rules of collaboration failed to prevent unequal influence in scientific exchange.[11] One factor that survived and surpassed the bureaucracy of the organization was experts.

Scholars continue to document the perspectives of developing countries whose expert scientists wished to join the WHO's international projects. Randall Packard recently pointed out the origins of the WHO's problem with achieving international teamwork. Apart from its obsession with magic-bullet solutions, its health interventions were largely developed outside of the countries where real problems existed, resulting in its ignorance of basic health services.[12] In the 1950s, during the first wave of scientific expertise, experts felt an imperative to explain how the sciences functioned without questioning their nature and methods of inquiry.[13] People largely assumed that science was true knowledge and technology was the foundation for progress. When WHO scientists looked for experts from other cultures, they naturally paid attention to those who looked like themselves. By doing so, they ignored a contributing factor that also shaped the agency of these non-Western experts from the perspective of participating countries. After World War II, the scientific community saw a sea change from what John Krige has called "inter-imperial networks" to a new social relation exemplified by Cold War rivalries and international collaboration.[14] From the perspective of developing countries, scientists' activities resembled Sunil Amrith's description of an "administrative pilgrimage" and the "self-fashioning" that occurred among scientists chronicled by Warwick Anderson and Hans Pols's relentless postcolonial critique of medicine and global health.[15] And even more recently, scholars of science, technology, and society have applied the image of a previously described "dreamscape" to explain Asian scientists' efforts toward modernization in the wake of infringement by Western powers.[16] These spaces include corporations, social movements, professional societies, and even different political entities where scientists were drawn to participate. For the WHO's member states, sending scientists to work at the headquarters in Geneva became an element of that dreamscape.

The WHO's social psychiatry project was not entirely consistent with its other organizational practices. The plan to survey mental illnesses, nationally and internationally, and to standardize classification was a multicenter effort. The WHO gathered and distributed expert consultants and the information they produced. Those experts then maintained a degree of teamwork as they developed instruments for use in underdeveloped countries. It is still debatable, however, whether the WHO's participating internationalists did eventually transform the psychiatric cultures in their countries of origin. As studies of global mental health have shown, the infrastructure for supporting mental health in many developing countries is still either inadequate or considerably different from the vision offered by Geneva. The WHO may have demonstrated the feasibility of international collaboration in psychiatric research, but local provisions for mental health still varied. The following activities of local experts outside Geneva demonstrate the commonality that facilitated the WHO's project.

Africa and Latin America

When the WHO first planned its mental health projects, Africa played a trivial role, at least in part because the pressing problem in much of the continent was infectious disease. In the decade after World War II, however, many areas in Africa belonging to the United Nations' category of "non-self-governing territories" under its trusteeship structure were still under the de facto colonization of European empires.[17] They were viewed as "tribal regions" isolated from modern medicine and ill equipped to apply psychiatric interventions.[18] An obvious voice for this view was the colonial psychiatrist J. C. Carothers (1903–1989). Born in South Africa, Carothers trained as a physician at St. Thomas Hospital in London but was almost self-taught in psychiatry. He spent two decades working in and reporting observations from Mathari Hospital and a prison in Nairobi, Kenya.[19] In 1952 he produced a report emphasizing the intellectual and cultural inferiority of his patients there, whose brain morphology and substandard morality, he claimed, represented the "African mind."[20] In the 1950s, despite ample criticism from anthropologists for ignoring modern studies on social organizations and for having a flawed research methodology, Carothers still received intellectual support from Margaret Mead and other WHO figures, who remained silent on his racist claims.[21]

With her notion of "one world, many cultures," Mead implied that culture was an external influence, not an intrinsic determinant of a population's mental capacity. Such an approach differed from mainstream psychiatry, then still under the influence of Emil Kraepelin. Despite stressing the importance of cross-national surveys, Kraepelin and many of his followers continued to affirm a biological—and, more precisely, a racialized—pathology of mental disorders. Culture, they thought, was a social determinant that could affect the clinical manifestations, disease patterns, and prognoses of mental disorders among the world's citizens. Survey studies of mental health in the early postwar period fell largely between the biological determinism represented by Carothers and the neutral mapping of different cultures. In the period of decolonization, therefore, social scientists studying Africa continued to emphasize cultural characteristics when documenting mental symptoms.[22]

Toward the end of the 1950s, mental health research in Africa underwent a sea change. More writers disparaged the nature of "African minds," which they claimed were structurally inferior to those of Caucasians.[23] Survey works on mental disorders, however, did not occur until 1959.[24] Yet several proto-epidemiological studies, based on Nigerian-born psychiatrist Thomas Adeoye Lambo's (1923–2004) observations in Aro Hospital in Nigeria, had already surveyed the symptomatology and incidence of psychiatric disorders, starting in 1955.[25] Lambo had completed his medical degree at the University of Birmingham in 1948, followed by specialty training in psychiatry in London at Maudsley Hospital with Aubrey Lewis, which shaped the perspective he took on the nature of mental disorders. He returned to Nigeria in 1954, becoming the superintendent of Aro Mental Hospital.

Like other experts whom the WHO consulted and who eventually sought a pilgrimage to Geneva, Lambo criticized the work of ethnopsychiatrists, including J. C. Carothers, as pseudo-scientific, racially biased, and misleading. In a report published in 1955, he said that much of ethnopsychiatry was "useful for the guidance of research, but containing so many obvious gaps and inconsistencies, giving rise to so many unanswerable questions, that [it] can no longer be seriously presented as valid observations of scientific merit."[26] Although trained in the West, Lambo collaborated with traditional healers, believing that in his own culture, traditional medical practitioners provided meaningful care for mentally ill patients. While practicing in his home country, he found that his fellow Nigerians suffered from high rates of depression and schizophrenia. To prove his argument, he designed comparative studies with other researchers.[27] Attempting to emancipate psychiatry in Nigeria from the bonds of colonial racialism, he sought international collaborators for cross-cultural research.[28] In 1961, together with Alexander Leighton (1908–2007), mastermind of the Stirling County Study in Canada, a well-known research program conducted in the mid-1950s that investigated the relations between sociocultural environment and mental illness,[29] Lambo embarked on the Cornell-Aro Mental Health Project. The study compared types and rates of mental illness in Yoruba communities in West Africa with mental illness in Canadians in North America, and so established methods for further investigations.

Lambo's unconventional work was published in 1960 as the monograph *Psychiatric Disorder among the Yoruba.*[30] Surprisingly, the team found that symptom prevalence and type among the Yoruba and the residents of Stirling County were curiously similar, leading to the conclusion that cultural differences may have been overemphasized. The team's work surely increased the visibility of Africa in the WHO's project, then still in the planning stage, and led to Ibadan, Nigeria, becoming a field research center (FRC) for the International Pilot Study of Schizophrenia. The legacy of Lambo's ambition to modernize African psychiatry, however, remains uneven. The World Mental Health Surveys conducted in the first decade of the twenty-first century, for example, revealed a much smaller percentage of Nigerians receiving treatment for mental health problems than people with comparable problems in other parts of the world. Apparently, inadequate recognition of psychiatric problems and lack of available services have persisted.[31] With the rise of global mental health campaigns, considerable attention is still paid to the lack of psychiatric resources in Africa.

Compared to Africa, Latin America offers a more complex history of mental health research and practice. It is, therefore, difficult to draw conclusions about the region's relationship with the WHO in the first ever International Social Psychiatry Project. The Latin American story, however, reveals the WHO's logic in recruiting experts: the WHO seemed to place more importance on ease of collaboration with local psychiatrists than on how significant their expertise was. This logic indirectly corroborated Tsung-yi Lin's theory that training was the main factor that facilitated collaboration.

Latin America was associated with the Pan American Health Organization at the very beginning of the twentieth century, but as a vast region with different levels of development, progress in public health was sporadic. As in Africa, mental health in Latin America was a new component of public health. Psychiatry, however, was not new. For example, starting in the first half of the twentieth century, and reacting to the crisis of positivism, the decline of authoritarian practices at universities, and the cultural impact of European immigration, Argentina became well known for its psychoanalytic culture.[32] And Hargreaves's speech in Buenos Aires in 1953 on his vision of cross-country comparative surveys immediately inspired the German-trained Argentine social psychiatrist Eduardo Krapf to share his similar vision.[33] After Krapf left for a teaching position at Leeds, the WHO soon recruited Hargreaves to head the mental health unit. Krapf led the unit's preparation for its international collaboration on social psychiatry and gained international prominence, though he never had much to do with transforming psychoanalytic practice in Argentina.

Argentina resisted German and French psychoanalytic theories that addressed inner psychic conflicts rather than external forces. This resistance was rooted in the country's traditional aversion to Western capitalist approaches to mental disorders. In the 1950s, Argentine psychiatrists began to argue for social factors in establishing the etiology of mental disorders, leading to conflict with those who assumed that intrinsic mechanisms caused psychiatric symptoms. Some Argentine psychoanalysts tried to trace the origin of social and economic problems to inner psychic factors; others attempted to develop psychoanalytic categories rooted in the nation's social and political issues. These debates led to extensive discussion about "external" factors on the therapeutic couch.[34] Despite their disputes, however, Argentine psychiatrists together disseminated psychoanalytic languages and methods, especially among nonspecialist middle-class groups who would play a central role in calling for social and political reform. In an authoritarian country, psychoanalytic theories became a refuge for left-wing scholars to conceal their political discontent.[35] Though psychiatric knowledge was evident from clinics to street corners, its appropriation in Argentina was idiosyncratic.

Also beginning in the 1960s, several mental health studies in Latin America piqued the interest of the international psychiatric community. However, the research was theoretically diverse and limited in size. For example, the Peruvian Ministry of Public Health and Social Assistance supported several studies to determine mental health conditions in and around Lima. They used the Cornell Medical Index to compare data collected in different areas and found rural populations relatively healthier than those who resided in the city. In addition to relying on epidemiology, scholars began to notice cultural aspects of mental illness among Andean populations.[36] McGill's journal *Transcultural Psychiatry* periodically featured small-scale Peruvian surveys that were anthropological, offering cultural explanations of behavior and mental disorders. The studies explored a range of topics from drinking to Peruvian family kinship personalities, such as those related to *susto*, a condition thought of as "soul abduction," which is now categorized as a culture-bound syndrome.[37] The close ties between Peruvian doctors and psychiatrists at McGill's transcultural psychiatry research unit have been maintained to the present day.

However, the WHO wanted more than just outstanding researchers. It sought scientists who were willing to cooperate with the research timeline and who could generate data that WHO officials thought came from a "suitable field" that could represent "the locals." Neither Buenos Aires nor Lima became a social psychiatry field research center. Following two seminars—one in Cuernavaca, Mexico, in 1962, and another in Buenos Aires, in 1963—the WHO aligned the objectives of mental health studies in Latin America with the objectives of the headquarters in Geneva. Mental health thus became a category within public health, and mental disorders became subject to prevention.[38] In the seminars, experts prioritized the investigation of psychiatric problems according to the percentage of the population affected and the extent to which their problems obstructed social and economic progress. In 1965, the social psychiatry project chose Santiago de Cali, in southwest Colombia, Latin America's third most populated country, for a field research center.

At the Universidad del Valle in Cali, Carlos A. León's work had not attracted the same attention as that of other experts, but he was the perfect choice for collaborating with the WHO possibly due to his similar training background. Born in Ecuador in 1926, León received his medical education at Pedro Carbo National College. After working a few years at San Lázaro mental health hospital in Quito, he went to Tulane University to further his study of psychiatry under the supervision of the controversial Robert D. Heath (1915–1999).[39] León chose Tulane because of its dual emphasis on psychoanalysis and biological psychiatry, which allowed him to pursue his original interest and new clinical methods. He began to teach at the Universidad del Valle in 1955. As a pioneering psychiatrist who wrote about *susto*, he applied sociocultural insights to understanding folk illnesses.[40] Still dissatisfied with his work and unhappy that psychiatric practice in Colombia

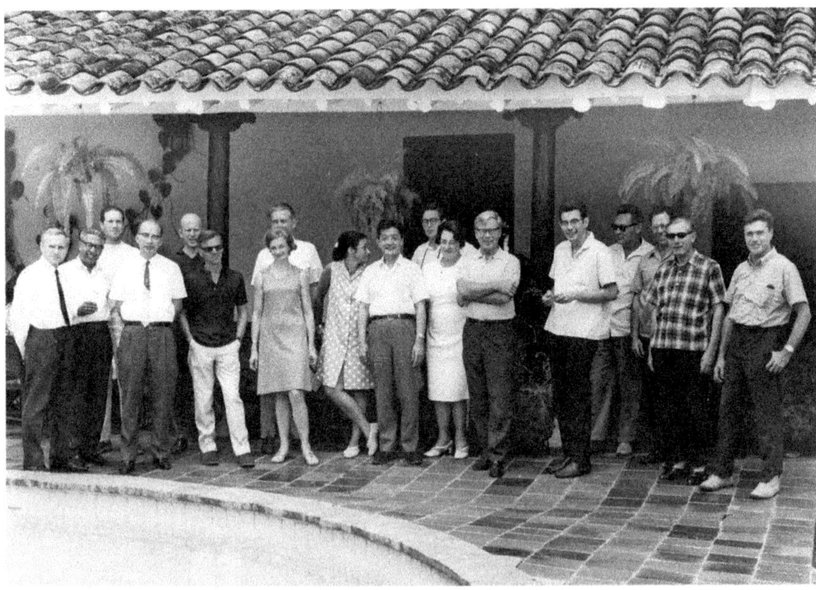

Figure 4.1
WHO's Mental Health team on their research trip in Cali, Colombia.
Credit: Eileen Brooke Papers. Queen Mary, University of London archives. AIMG-0802.

was primarily limited to long confinements in mental health hospitals, he returned to Tulane as a full-time student and obtained a master's degree in epidemiology from its school of public health, which had a long tradition of applying preventive approaches to tropical medicine.[41] Upon his return to Cali, León began to study the problem of mental disorders through epidemiological efforts.[42] When Cali was chosen by the WHO to be a field research center, it was in transition from an agricultural to an industrial city and was about to enter a period of peace after a series of struggles between the country's two leading political parties.[43] Its young population and influx of migrants displayed characteristics typical of change in developing countries.

Taiwan: The Ideal Bedfellow

As the WHO sought collaborating countries that could fully engage with the agenda set in Geneva, the choice of Taiwan was very different from the cases of Africa and Latin America. Taiwan became an ideal participant to represent the Western Pacific not least because Tsung-yi Lin came to head the social psychiatry project. Lin had trained to become a psychiatrist in Tokyo during the war and gained insight into cross-cultural psychiatric studies from his mentor, Yushi Uchimura (1897–1980). In 1955, when Ronald Hargreaves had a layover in Taipei, en route from a regional conference of the WHO's Western Pacific regional office in Manila, he met Lin, then head of psychiatry at National Taiwan University Hospital. According to Lin's recollection, they met at the airport, and Hargreaves was holding Lin's paper from the journal *Psychiatry*. Hargreaves praised the paper highly and immediately invited him to become a consultant for the WHO.[44] The story implies a meeting of minds between the WHO and Lin, whose work did indeed offer potential for collaboration. The emergence of this young and previously unknown psychiatrist within the clique of renowned internationalists, however, required other factors, which eventually propelled Lin toward becoming the medical officer overseeing the WHO's first social psychiatry project.

Lin's report in *Psychiatry*, "A Study of the Incidence of Mental Disorder in Chinese and Other Cultures," analyzed a survey of three Chinese townships with communities of different socioeconomic levels and four aboriginal communities with various degree of "acculturation." Lin and his team concluded that the prevalence of mental disorders across these communities was the same.[45] This series of surveys, the first of its kind in Taiwan, was glorified as the first "Chinese" psychiatric population study to gain international attention. The paper also opened a channel between Geneva and Asia. In the book *Psychiatry around the Globe*, Julian Leff (1938–), who was later involved in the International Pilot Study of Schizophrenia at the WHO, identified flaws in Lin's research design regarding sex and age correction in statistics,[46] but despite the critique, Lin and his team had

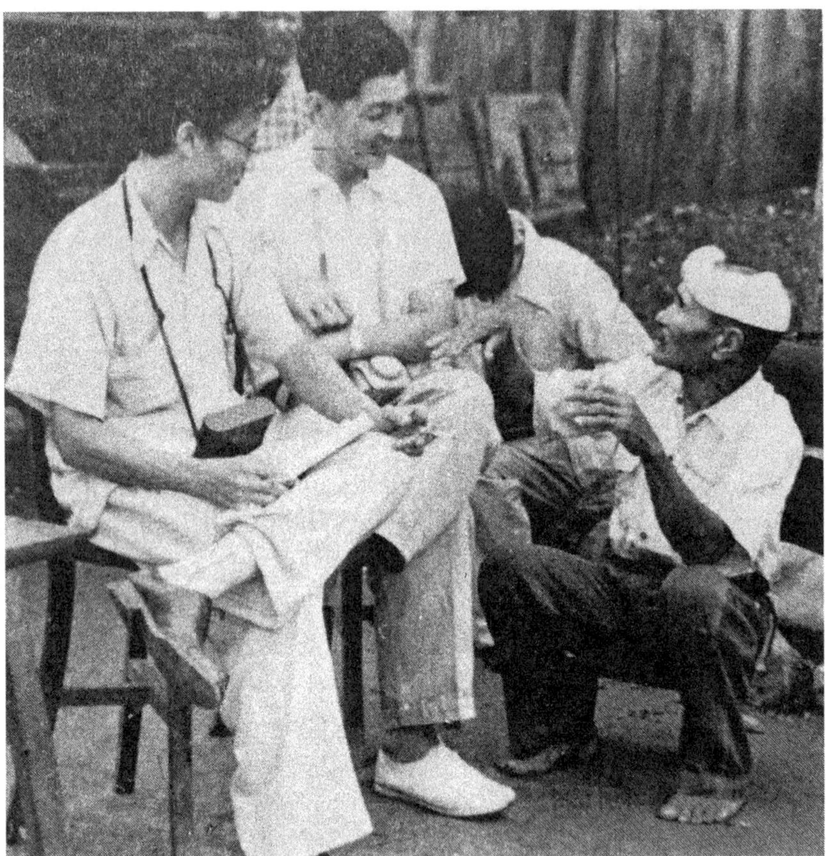

Figure 4.2
Tsung-yi Lin and Hsien Rin conducting mental health surveys in Taiwan villages, 1946–1948.
Source: Marnie Copland, *A Lin Odyssey* (New Orleans: Paraclete Press, 1987), 106.

charted a path for transnational research that would inform the WHO's social psychiatry projects and facilitate collaboration between Geneva and an underdeveloped "non-West."

Incomplete Decolonization

Many factors pushed Lin's work onto the international stage, but the relationship between the WHO and Taiwan was more than a marriage of convenience. Rather, it reflected the rise of scientific internationalism—an aspiration to develop a model of collaboration—and a common language of psychiatry that was free of racial prejudice. As chapter 3 explained, decentralization and outsourcing at the WHO invited a diverse range of participants and promoted an optimism for effective collaboration to understand shared disease profiles in modern psychiatry.[47] As global developmentalism in the postwar period transformed the contact zone between the West and non-West, scientific views of race underwent an epistemological transition from biological determinism to neo-Freudian theory.[48] This turn, however, depended on a legacy of colonial science: categories of mental illness, survey methods, and images of populations unsupported by scientific evidence. More recent psychopathological theories and research methods have also challenged claims that the human sciences have been successfully deracialized in the post-genomic era.

In fact, the WHO's social psychiatry project never fully rejected race as an analytic category, despite the effort of international organizations (e.g., UNESCO).[49] Race emerged as a cultural sticking point among participating member states, reflecting Margaret Mead's "one world, many cultures." As medical historians of culture and colonialism have shown, racial science continued to influence psychiatry, with concepts rooted in colonial experience. At the WHO, despite support for decolonization, Hargreaves sought to scale up Emil Kraepelin's cross-cultural survey on mental illness, despite Kraepelin's notions of racial hierarchy, and Lin's community surveys built on ethnographic data acquired during the Japanese colonial period. Lin's work also relied heavily on the household registration system left behind by the Japanese colonial administration, which became the sine qua non for researchers dealing with limited resources and postwar devastation.

In his memoir, Lin recollected that, before his work, modern psychiatry had been a "barren desert" in Taiwan, although it had been developing in the region for more than a decade under Japanese rule.[50] Colonial administration in Taiwan, as in other colonies in Asia, applied racial science to define native diseases.[51] Colonial psychiatry presumed that there were distinct mental disorders in racially defined populations. In Taiwan, medical practice before and during World War II was marked by the identification of ethnically understood mental illnesses.[52] The Japanese administration used these diseases, together with other biomedical discourses, to define national characteristics, which in turn grounded psychiatric treatment in assumptions of innate difference and provided a biological foundation for colonial power. The notion of nationally identifiable mental illnesses receded at the end of Japanese colonial rule, but the idea had informed psychiatric institutions during a crucial period of Taiwanese medicine.

The ethnopsychiatry developed in Japan and Taiwan differed somewhat from the racial science that had developed in tandem with European imperial expansion, however. In Africa and South Asia, for example, ethnopsychiatry emerged in response to encounters between colonizers and colonized, becoming part of the regulatory power of empires. Yet in Taiwan, colonial psychiatry was developed to inform the colonial government, with surveys used as part of a knowledge-based development strategy.[53] Even so, Japan had been influenced by the West, particularly Germany, since the 1870s, and Japanese psychiatry before and during World War II was thus a combination of German medical science and Japanese tradition.[54] In prewar Taiwan, the human sciences showcased Japan as a scientifically advanced modern state. The culture of institutionalizing mentally ill patients in Japan and its colonies provided suitable samples for psychiatrists to conduct catchment studies based on statistical science.[55] Survey studies used in psychiatry, as in many other disciplines, served both scientific and colonial interests. Psychiatry thus served the Japanese government's agenda. Not long before the Asian Pacific War, epidemiological studies of mental disorders were also conducted by doctors working for Taihoku Imperial University on Hainan Island.[56] They were but one area of preparation for Japan's short-lived attempt to form the Greater East Asia Co-Prosperity Sphere, an economic and military bloc consisting of countries within East and Southeast Asia aligned against Western colonization. Unlike colonial psychiatric theories developed mainly in Europe, in Japanese studies human subjects were assumed to be biologically equal, even if culturally different.[57] This view of human distinction, which grew from an empirical foundation established during Japanese colonial rule, affected psychiatry's later development in Taiwan. When Tsung-yi Lin became the first director of the psychiatric department at National Taiwan University Hospital (NTUH), he reviewed the records left by the Japanese and used them, together with his own research, to contribute to the establishment of psychiatry in decolonized (and "re-Sinicized") Taiwan.

The Japanese survey-based approach to science, with a traceable Kraepelinian genealogy, influenced the first large-scale investigation of mental illnesses in Taiwan. In Japan, Lin had trained in psychiatry at the University of Tokyo and at Mazusawa Hospital; Mazusawa's psychiatric department was headed by Yushi Uchimura, who had studied in Germany under Emil Kraepelin.[58] At Mazusawa, Uchimura adopted German research methods to measure the burden of mental disease in different populations. In conducting large-scale surveys, he constructed a theory for the interpretation of psychiatric illnesses within a Darwinian evolutionary framework. Uchimura argued that psychiatry can extend research and services to populations that are incompletely developed (as he believed children and women were) by elucidating the psychopathology of "primitive" people.[59] With a survey in Hokkaido, for example, he identified several psychiatric reactions in the indigenous Ainu community that he defined as racially determined.[60]

Whether Lin directly employed Uchimura's Darwinian framework in his own surveys is unclear, but his team adopted Uchimura's survey method. When Lin was studying in Tokyo, apart from Uchimura's supervision, he was also greatly influenced by books such as Dugald Christie's *Thirty Years in Moukden* and Herbert Day Lamson's *Social Pathology in China*, which influenced his thinking on the relationship between physical and mental disorders and the social conditions among Chinese populations.[61] To develop psychiatric services in Taiwan, he acquired data on the size of the affected population and the prevalence of mental disorders. In 1946, he mobilized the local gentry, elders, and police to facilitate investigation of the distribution of psychiatric diseases in Baksa, a town in northern Taiwan. To reduce costs, he employed the *hokō* system, the Japanese mechanism of community-based law enforcement and civil control.[62] In this system, set up by the colonial government to enforce compliance, a neighborhood leader was responsible for a group of households, ensuring that they paid taxes, supplied labor for state projects, and participated in public health campaigns. Lin's team relied on the *hokō* leaders to survey three Chinese townships with various levels of socioeconomic status. Together with his survey of 19,931 Chinese individuals, his 1953 publication documented varied cultures, lifestyles, and quantifiable class differences, which served as parameters for differentiation in survey samples.

Interestingly, the NTUH team first investigated the dominant Han Chinese and other ethnic groups in Taiwan, but a shortage of background data compelled the survey team to refer to Japanese colonial research. Investigative reports published by the Japanese in the early twentieth century, and later published in five volumes as *Report on Investigations into the Customs of Aboriginal Peoples*, provided information about the traditions of Taiwan's indigenous tribes, including material culture, lifestyle, and descriptions of psychiatric diseases. The report was the outcome of a survey that spanned more than a decade and provided the groundwork for lawmaking in the colony. Much of the team's foundational work was based on surveys conducted by Japanese colonial authorities.

Between 1946 and 1948, Lin and his students combined the Japanese results and the research framework used to study the Han Chinese. Between 1949 and 1953, Hsien Rin (1925–2016), a student of Lin, used similar methods to survey 11,442 people from four indigenous groups. Rin and his colleagues sought support from influential community leaders, who assisted them in identifying sites for study.[63] In the field, a community leader accompanied investigators (psychiatrists, students, and nurses) on household visits and assisted in securing interviews by explaining the purpose of the visits and acting as interpreters. Community mediation led to considerable data on mental illnesses in these groups.[64] Like his teacher Lin, Rin began his research assuming that ethnic groups exhibit distinct patterns related to mental health problems, but statistical results instead indicated similarities between the groups. Similar lifetime prevalence rates were evident for all mental disorders identified among the Chinese (9.4 per 1,000) and indigenous populations (9.5 per 1,000). The rates for psychotic disorders were also nearly identical (3.9 per 1,000 for Chinese and 3.8 per 1,000 for indigenous Taiwanese).[65] The team concluded that aborigines were not necessarily mentally healthier, at least according to the prevalence of mental illness. The researchers did observe lower rates of schizophrenic symptoms among indigenous groups, but they speculated that the difference might be the result of proportionally larger numbers of deaths among indigenous schizophrenic patients because of their limited ability to adjust to stress and deprivation during World War II. Like the Japanese, the researchers categorized ethnic groups according to differing degrees of acculturation. Yet they also avoided predominant anthropological theories that differentiated racial hierarchies, and instead simply assumed that different mental diseases were biologically determined in different races that possessed different mental capacities. The research findings reported by Tsung-yi Lin and his students laid the foundation for his participation in Hargreaves's "manageable project" a decade later. Their methods thus continued to inform the WHO's social psychiatry project.

Chinese as Scientific Other

Another factor contributing to Lin's involvement with the WHO's project was the scientific stance of his country's psychiatrists, which corresponded with dominant views in Geneva. From the founding of the League of Nations through the interwar period, experts from the Global South had been theoretically treated as equals. After World War II, the WHO's expanding mission maintained roles for experts from all over the globe, while modern psychiatry simultaneously sought to establish itself as an autonomous scientific discipline among other medical specialties. At the closing period of the war, scientists in Taiwan embraced a doctrine of modern medicine that subordinated experts' own ethnic identities and rooted scientific inquiry in universal humanism and rationality.[66] In postwar Taiwan, this position supported the development of a scientific discipline in the decolonizing state.

Psychiatrists in Taiwan had to develop their professional influence in a state with limited resources. Researchers wanted to apply their Japanese medical education, conduct research on a national scale, and identify differences among their patients, but as Tsung-yi Lin recalled in his memoir, an updated survey had identified only 819 mentally ill patients when he assumed his post in 1948 at NTUH.[67] Furthermore, Japanese psychiatrists had been repatriated immediately after the war, leaving approximately 300 patients without care and only one Japanese psychiatrist to handle the handover. National Taiwan University then replaced Taihoku Imperial University as the hospital affiliated with psychiatry,[68] and Lin had to operate an understaffed department with insufficient support from the new government. At age twenty-six, he returned to his homeland to develop modern psychiatry for Chinese people, a project that reflected the objectives of decolonization and national autonomy. And government officials took mental illness and the influence of the colonial medical paradigm seriously. NTUH Psychiatric Department case files documented a rapid increase in immigrant Chinese outpatients seeking psychiatric help and indicated that some had developed mental illnesses.

Lin's motivation to conduct an epidemiological survey was multifold. He recalled initially wanting to study the profiles of mental illnesses among his fellow Chinese.[69] As a child, he had been confused about whether his name was Japanese (Hayashi) or Chinese (Lin) because the Chinese characters for the Japanese name Hayashi and the Chinese name Lin are the same. But as an adult, he had identified as Chinese in response to Japanese colonialism, and his father had encouraged him to study Chinese psychology. Differences between the Chinese and Lin's own identity also motivated his research. In his postwar encounters with newly arrived immigrants from mainland China, he had noted psychological manifestations that failed to conform to his expectations. Conflicts between these immigrants and indigenous Taiwanese further piqued his interest in the ethnic roots of behavior.

The psychiatrists who conducted survey studies in Taiwan engaged in meticulous data collection. They not only applied existing classifications of mental disorders but also continuously identified symptoms that represented culture-bound syndromes. While studying mental illness among Chinese populations in Taiwan, Lin first observed a rare convulsive hysteria and then discovered several culture-bound syndromes prevalent in the Chinese population. One was *hsieh-ping*, or "devil's sickness," which was characterized by a trancelike state in which the patient identified with a dead person and spoke in a strange tone of voice, mostly about ancestor worship, from thirty minutes to several hours. The syndrome occurred frequently among highly religious people. Symptoms included tremors, disorientation, delirium, and occasional visual or auditory hallucinations, and resembled the possession phenomenon identified in Japan as *kitsunetsuki*, or "fox possession."[70]

From the closing decades of the nineteenth century to the early twentieth century, similar phenomena to *kitsunetsuki* had been observed in Taiwan as a case of a native neurosis. It had been reported in the *Bulletin of Taiwan Medical Affairs*, providing one of the main reports of culture-bound syndromes identified by psychiatrists in East Asia.[71] The writers of this report believed that the subject's development of possession-like symptoms resembled the psychiatric manifestation observed by Uchimura in the Ainu community. Other examples included the *utox* reaction among the Atayal in Taiwan, *imu* among the Ainu in Japan, and *koro* in various Southeast Asian countries.[72] Apart from the *utox* reaction observed in the Atayal tribe, Lin identified few cases among indigenous peoples that could be classified as psychoneurosis, and he maintained that the symptomology of *utox* was determined culturally rather than racially. Overall, results indicated the universality of mental illnesses among various populations, and the research team concluded that culturally bound syndromes shared a similar underlying psychopathology, triggered by stress and fear.

Taiwan as an International Laboratory to Understand the "Chinese"

In early post-World War II Taiwan, Chinese populations were convenient subjects for the World Health Organization, even though the island's area comprised only 0.37% that of the mainland, which by the early 1950s was behind the "iron curtain" of communism.[73] Under Chiang Kai-shek's control, Taiwan, together with Hong Kong, became substitutes for scholars eager to learn about China. Deemed "free China," the region eventually filled China's seat at the UN, despite some calling this "an absurdity" (see chapter 1).[74] As a civilization acounting for more than one-fifth of the world's population, China was one of the three UN member states that first proposed the establishment of the WHO. Taiwan, however, came to represent China and became the laboratory for international organizations seeking to understand Chinese culture and to apply global developmentalism to Chinese society.

Taiwan was a site for most of the WHO's projects, among them interventions in nursing and mother-child relationships as well as trachoma prevention. Most notable was its participation in the Malaria Eradication Program (MEP), launched in 1955. With Taiwanese moderniziation—especially the health infrastructure established by Japan, the Rockefeller Foundation's vested interest in the late 1940s, and the island's militarization in the postwar period—Taiwan had successfully eradicated malaria by 1965.[75] Taiwan was thus prominent in global development when the WHO was recruiting participants for its mental health projects, and it became the second-ranked member state to Australia while project leaders were prioritizing countries for collaboration. China's representative at the WHO had been Yü-Lin Ch'eng, the founder of Nanjing Brain Hospital, who had been educated at Peking

Union Hospital. He joined the expert committee of the WHO's Mental Health Unit, but when the Western Pacific regional office was relocated from Shanghai to Manila, he moved to Taiwan and practiced at a veterans hospital, before eventually landing in the United States until retirement.

Dreamscape of Experts

The WHO's system of expert consultants recruited worldwide talent to Geneva but needed to entice psychiatrists from developing countries to join a project few fully understood. The WHO had a limited budget, a peculiar working environment, and an agenda still in progress. Before Lin relocated to the WHO headquarters, other experts had refused the invitation. Eduardo Krapf, for example, turned down Hargreaves's offer, citing family concerns. As historians have noted, a sense of "administrative pilgrimage" had led countries to send expert consultants to international health organizations in the interwar period.[76] The WHO's outsourcing strategy, in contrast, identified and prioritized health concerns in developing countries, including China. Underdeveloped countries were eager to send specialists to the WHO to acquire expertise, while the organization recognized these same specialists as experts and aspired to learn from them. Those trained in scientifically advanced countries regarded themselves as equal to their counterparts in Europe, Japan, and North America.

After World War II, "national self-fashioning" among scientists was essential to facilitating collaboration with Geneva.[77] Not only could colleagues communicate internationally, but the WHO provided a powerful catalyst for countries to represent themselves through science and medicine in the Cold War world order. Most East Asian intellectuals had viewed Japan as their model for modernization, but with decolonization, the WHO became the platform for developing their expertise. Tsung-yi Lin's enthusiasm for the WHO was thus an element of what Sheila Jasanoff and Sang-Hyun Kim call "the dreamscape."[78] His research may have had statistical flaws and lacked attention to the effects of age and gender, but he was willing to relocate and anxious to convince the WHO that Taiwan could make a substantial contribution.

The relationship between the WHO's Mental Health Unit and developing countries was not exactly a "trading zone" of science cooperation, however, in which the stakeholders in an international project agreed on rules of collaboration.[79] Most developing countries that sent experts had no cross-border communication with each other, and experts spoke different languages and had different cultural experiences. Nonetheless, these participants arrived at the WHO through similar channels, had received similar training in modern psychiatry, and shared a similar vision for a global comparative study of mental disorders that would establish universal diagnostic criteria. The Mental Health Unit could not have been successful without a shared ethos among WHO participants and core staff. Lin's research received considerable attention because it was an epidemiological study using rigorous survey methods in a developing country that the WHO had prioritized as a beneficiary of aid.

In 1964, Lin was appointed a medical officer in the WHO's Mental Health Section. His proposed International Social Psychiatry Project on psychiatric epidemiology and social psychiatry, with its four programs, together with the International Pilot Study of Schizophrenia (IPSS), later confirmed the universal profile of schizophrenia and led to the first international epidemiological study on schizophrenia and the first recognized psychiatric classification system.[80] It required new statistical methods and computing capabilities, including programs like CATEGO (see chapter 5), which would categorize large amounts of data collected globally. Lin had been unfamiliar with these methods, and his pilot study on schizophrenia was criticized for its sampling and data correction. Moreover, schizophrenia was only one disease validated with epidemiological data in the fifth chapter of the *ICD*, and it, too, was subsequently deemed flawed. Nevertheless, Lin and other psychiatrists at the WHO established a professional community through a global network that included developing countries as participants. Their work attracted leading theorists and self-fashioned experts who were competent within the WHO-designed domain. Their involvement enabled them to produce policy-relevant knowledge.

Imagined Equal Footing

The partnership between the WHO and its member states was dynamic, the result of the mutual imagination of experts from the organization and developing countries, and it strengthened international collaboration in science. The WHO's technical assistance design originally avoided becoming overly instructive. It mapped out an ideal world, in which experts coming from member states, despite their differences in previous international exposure, enjoyed equal opportunities to communicate, exchange ideas, and eventually work on a project together. In reality, however, members' degree of decolonization and development differed, and Geneva's treatment of developing countries was influenced by their colonial pasts. We can now see the distance between the idealism of the WHO's social psychiatry project, based on the concept of world citizenship, and its uneven application across participating countries. The WHO's brain drain of experts from some participating states failed to alter their psychiatric cultures fully, and today, as a "gold standard" of mental illness, the refined *ICD* may still have difficulties adopting the WHO system.

Despite these imperfections, scientific projects at the local and global levels informed and transformed one another. In an atmosphere of postwar scientific internationalism, with the foundations of a new world order codified and promoted by the United Nations, new measures of investigation emerged. A mutual vision of the prospects for science propelled collaboration among psychiatrists at the WHO and in collaborating countries, and that vision established a common platform to facilitate international science. Experts recruited by the WHO, despite their varied origins, appeared relatively homogeneous not because of their cultural backgrounds but due to their training. They bore a similar intellectual genealogy inherited from a handful of schools of epidemiological thought or from collaboration with research teams experienced in cross-cultural surveys. Such intellectual similarity enabled them to communicate effectively and efficiently, and yet it also led them to ignore chances to see diseases in a different light in the still heterogeneous world for which the WHO originally stood.

Problems continued to emerge during the Cold War period, but the WHO remained committed to its search for data to support and optimize its standardized diagnostic criteria for mental disorders. In the case of Tsung-yi Lin, coming from Taiwan, an intended beneficiary as a developing country and a stand-in for China, the medical officer fit all practical roles in one. From a close-up examination of Taiwan, we see a *histoire croisée* of the WHO's International Social Psychiatry Project and its participating countries that relied on at least four contingencies. First, despite its postcolonial promise, the project could draw on concepts, methods, and survey studies of mental illness dating from the colonial past. Second, toward the end of World War II, scientists in Taiwan had established a scientific stance toward the Chinese that led researchers to conduct a survey study of mental illness among the Chinese and other populations. Third, though a small island a hundred miles off the southeastern coast of China, Taiwan became a laboratory for scientists seeking to apprehend Chinese society, as mainland China remained inaccessible during several decades of the Cold War. Fourth, psychiatrists from developing countries, Lin among them, pursued a dreamscape of modernization in the postwar world order in which they could represent their own modern nation-states within the structure of international organizations.

Tsung-yi Lin left halfway through the International Social Psychiatry Project, in 1969, but the work he had initiated continued. Internationalists at the WHO continued to pursue the model of international science, which Lin had helped to institutionalize. In 1973, when the United Nations General Assembly voted to replace Taiwan with the People's Republic of China as the official representative of China, the WHO continued to support Taiwan in its social psychiatric research. Here science prevailed over politics for a time. In Taiwan, Lin was praised as a pioneer of psychiatry, but many of his students abandoned his methods. Some pursued a cultural psychiatry that emphasized the local context of diseases and mental symptoms and, like psychiatrists in Argentina, developed an alternative discourse distinct from the state-sanctioned norm. In the 1970s, however, "global" and "local" scientists, the strange bedfellows who had been dreaming differently, began to develop disparate approaches. Croatian psychiatrist Norman Sartorius succeeded Lin to lead the mental health division of the organization and was celebrated as the major advocate of the WHO's social psychiatry project and its classification of mental disorders. Sartorius followed a career path similar to those of other experts in the organization. Even though he was educated in communist Yugoslavia, a country that was initially isolated from international society in the early postwar period, he was also devastated by war, discontented with the state of the discipline at home, and trained further at Maudsley.[81] By this time, however, the organization's operation had matured and could function smoothly, with a consistent structure and ideology, no matter who led the work. But the projects developed thereafter were less innovative. Perhaps this shift explains why the contemporary movement in global mental health was initiated by another group of thinkers.

5 Technology

The 1950s and 1960s were the age of diagnosis in the history of psychiatry.[1] Globally, this development depended on technology. During this period, responding to rampant infectious diseases, the notion of technical assistance accelerated the application of quick-fix solutions to complex problems. This aspiring, "can do" optimism encouraged public health planners to believe that they were capable of rapidly transforming societies in the world.[2] In the field of mental health, it was also through technology that mental disorders were finally made visible, measurable, and eventually manageable. Advances in videotaping, international communication, data sciences, and the methods of standardization all shaped the metrics for classifying mental disorders at the international level. In the hub of transcultural psychiatry, Eric Wittkower noted, "Technological advance, the ease of travel, combined with an awareness of the interdependence of the world in the nuclear age, has brought psychiatrists face to face with psychological problems in other countries."[3] At the WHO, the International Social Psychiatry Project reflected shared values among visionary thinkers working within a robust organization. Guided by the notion of world citizenship, WHO experts sought standard metrics to identify symptoms and diseases worldwide. But their efforts could not be fulfilled without turning to technology. That technology augmented human judgment and supported the project's scale and scope.

Before detailing the use of technology, we need to look at the concept of standardization. Why were standardized metrics so important? Historians of science are familiar with how standardization from the early modern period onward played a part in the creation of a republican polity, how it accelerated the flow of commerce, facilitated scientific communication, and prevented hazards in naval activities.[4] Today, the question is about the balance between the need for international comparability and official national statistics. But a half-century ago, international comparisons were an urgent goal for the scientists at the WHO. The United Nations and its specialized agencies played crucial roles in standardizing and coordinating international data complications.[5] They laid the foundations for standard definitions of diseases and common terminologies derived from commonly apprehended theoretical frameworks.

In mental health, the WHO's promotion of world citizenship was the guiding concept that directed the collection of data and the development of a uniform system for classifying disease. People came to the rapidly growing WHO in droves from various parts of the world to work together there and produce knowledge that promoted standard practices worldwide, fulfilling the WHO's ethos of "the highest attainable level of health for all people." The organization's decentralized structure—which extended to recruiting staff, collecting information, and planning projects—shaped its priorities. Historians have commented extensively about the ways the WHO's projects were either facilitated or hampered by its structure.[6] The organization was unique, and its broad scope and internal arrangements affected the production of scientific knowledge.

Creating standardized metrics was not a new task for an organization already experienced in dealing with epidemics of infectious disease.[7] Mental health, however, had just become an accepted field of public health, and producing metrics for mental health was difficult. One impediment was the variety of languages used among member states. Visual representation, enhanced by innovative technologies, could be used to facilitate communication; yet, in the early postwar period, psychiatrists tended to see modern technology as a source of mental disturbance rather than a means for medical advancement. Not until the mid-1960s did scientists rely on the mechanical hardware they had originally feared. This shift represented a technological turn.

Building Internationalism

Upon its establishment in 1948, the WHO was housed at the Palais des Nations, the Geneva headquarters of the United Nations. In 1959, the World Health Assembly decided to construct a new building to accommodate the growing organization. After an international competition, the Swiss architect

Jean Tschumi (1904–1962), whose work was influenced by the modernist movement, was selected to design the new headquarters. Located at the end of Avenue Appia, the new building, an iconic example of the International Style of architecture, was a vast multilevel block containing same-sized cells designed to maximize its function. The rooms were furnished with similar basic, multipurpose facilities, convenient for cross-sectional communication. Like other buildings in this style, this new structure promoted a city within a city, with citizens coming from all over the world to address similar objectives. In the foyer was a travel agency serving officers and consultants. The canteen provided world cuisines to a range of employees.

The building and its activities symbolized the infrastructure of the WHO's numerous megaprojects, and the functional complex conveyed the interests of internationalists in global health and beyond. The organization sought to resemble its aspiration of world citizenship, which became the leverage point for mobilizing scientists worldwide to collaborate. Knowledge making then required a rapidly growing staff and processes for managing information and expediting workflow. In 1964, while the WHO officially commenced its International Social Psychiatry Project, scientific technologies promoted numerically informed rationality and led to the development of abundant statistical technologies.

Together with the emergence of technology, standardization became a strategy for participants from various locations and disciplines to address the organization's programmatic goals. At the organization's inception, the Interim Commission established the Expert Committee of Biological Standardization to coordinate the standardization of diagnoses and treatment methods, vaccination processes, nutrient levels, use of antibiotics, and other concerns.[8] Mental health became part of this pervasive effort. Standardizing professional language, methods of data collection, and diagnostic criteria for mental disorders was a pressing need for the WHO, but a project of this scope required new technology. Expertise in mental health thus intersected with the new machinery of public health, transforming the values of world citizenship into an instrumental pursuit of standardized metrics.

Classification as Standardization

To facilitate a huge collaborative project, the WHO needed a set of agreed-upon rules that could apply across field sites. The process for developing norms at the WHO remains unclear, but as historical cases have shown, successful implementation was contingent on several factors, among them the WHO's bureaucracy, which had muted the idealism and hope that prevailed at the end of World War II. To recruit a staff committed to world citizenship, decision makers turned to informal processes. Rather than recruiting through official medical journals or newsletters, program directors asked researchers they knew to make personal recommendations. Information moved through interpersonal circles. The WHO thus recruited like-minded individuals, whose vision aligned with headquarters and whose backgrounds, ideologies, and professional practices were compatible with those in charge.

A chaotic classification of mental disorders hampered not only the implementation of mental health projects but also the development of standards. To conduct epidemiological studies, therefore, international collaborators sought standard diagnostic criteria. By the mid-1960s, the *ICD* system, with mental disorders included, had gone through three revisions. *ICD* was considered a model for designing global information schemes, despite uncertainty, ambiguity, and the practicalities of data quality.[9] In the 1960s, psychiatrists worldwide praised the decision to revise the *ICD*'s chapter on mental disorders. Before the WHO's Mental Health Unit proposed a revision, a truly world-recognized version of classification had been unavailable. Calling on experts they knew, members of the *ICD* working group applied the WHO's operational processes to gather comments on drafts. They held seminars in different parts of the world and involved psychiatrists from different regions. Researchers with experience developing disease profiles sought to devise a standard interviewing instrument for collecting as many symptoms as possible.

Numerical thinking was an important part of the WHO's project. While mental health experts, influenced by the promise of technology, prepared to revise the *ICD* system, they discussed whether the glossary of mental disorders should be replaced by codes.[10] In the end, even though the idea was not adopted, the instrumental rationality of numbers still permeated the WHO's entire International Social Psychiatry Project. In 1965, the project began its four stages. The first two—to standardize psychiatric diagnoses, classification, and statistics and to determine whether comparable cases of mental disorders could be identified across populations internationally—ran concurrently. The third part of the project was a longitudinal international epidemiological study focusing on a single disorder, schizophrenia, while the fourth stage was to devise and implement an international training program in social psychiatry. The Social Psychiatry Project stemmed from the WHO's recognition that epidemiological studies could play an important role in preventing and controlling mental disorders.

The Mental Health Unit's work and its Social Psychiatry Project on the revision of the *ICD* system raised a range of related questions for today's analysts: What did classification and standards achieve? Who did the work? How did collaboration happen? How was such a large-scale effort mobilized and accelerated? In the early twentieth century, anthropologists had studied classification as a stratagem for analyzing cultures deemed primitive and subject to Western colonial power, whereas in the postwar era, standardized measures were sought to inform a more unified world in which we evaluate ourselves. Psychiatrists saw the work on the *ICD* as crucial and imperative, but comments on the revision reflected both heterogeneity in representing disease and ignorance of local norms. For example, participating psychiatrists debated the inclusion of neurasthenia, a popular diagnosis for a kind of neurosis characterized by fatigue and some physical and emotional disturbances. Psychiatrists also had differing views on problematic drinking and what should be considered excessive consumption of alcohol, noting that excessive consumption in the United States might not be considered excessive in France.[11] Debates were fierce on diagnoses related to sexuality, such as homosexuality, erotomania, nymphomania, fetishism, pedophilia, transvestitism, exhibitionism, and mixed sexual deviation.[12] Several comments indicated psychiatrists' hesitation about the revision: they welcomed the new glossary of diagnoses, but many were concerned that the haste to complete it could limit close study and existing glossaries and their application. For example, Eric Stengel expressed to the project coordinator, Tsung-yi Lin, "If the International Glossary is meant to make National Glossaries unnecessary, which I suppose is its ultimate purpose, it will be essential for certain national peculiarities of classification to be referred to."[13]

Information Technology

One core value that mobilized the WHO's work on mental health was linking the epidemiology of mental health with that of public health, which would help elevate psychiatry to the status of a hard science and a medical specialty. The WHO's information transmission was unique in the way that technology was used to enhance the gathering and distribution of knowledge at a truly global level. To facilitate the transmitting of epidemiological data among participating countries, the WHO turned to the existing radio-telegraphing system. This information service for epidemiological data had been proposed and developed by the League of Nations during the interwar period. The system was created to communicate complete, reliable, and up-to-date information about infectious diseases between Geneva and the League's member states. Since the 1920s, the Epidemiological Intelligence station in Singapore had played an important role in collecting and broadcasting disease summaries between Asia and Europe. However, the service focused only on infectious diseases and did not cross the Atlantic.

By the 1950s, new and upgraded machinery was enhancing the compilation, transmission, and reception of epidemiological data against the backdrop of the Cold War. In 1951, a new Epidemiological Intelligence Service was created in the United States at the Communicable Disease Center (now known as the Centers for Disease Control and Prevention). Initially propelled forward by the Korean War and Cold War fears that the Communist bloc might deploy biological weapons in an attack on the United States, the EIS grew to become among the best known of the CDC's swiftly multiplying operations.[14] In 1957, the USSR launched the first artificial satellite, Sputnik-1, from the Baikonur Cosmodrome; orbiting the Earth in ninety-six minutes, Sputnik-1 could provide signals anywhere in its orbit. The UN turned to the International Telegraph Union (ITU), which had existed for a century, as its specialized agency in telecommunication. A main task of the newly restructured ITU was to develop recommendations for the standardization of telecommunicating equipment, systems, networks, and services.[15] By the late 1950s, the WHO's quarantine intelligence and information services brought together units in Geneva, Singapore, Washington, and Alexandria. The radio-telegraphic system in the western Pacific was networked through twelve stations across the Indian Ocean.

In mental health, these technologies were new. Toward the end of the nineteenth century, when Kraepelin embarked on his grand study of mental disorders in Southeast Asia, he operated as an old-fashioned ethnographer, documenting "undiscovered" cultures. But by 1964, while the WHO mental health experts were planning the International Social Psychiatry Project, new technological infrastructure offered international communication in real time. Households worldwide, for example, watched the Olympic Games held in Tokyo on television, and within a few years people watched Neil Armstrong's moon walk in real time. The WHO could now synchronize the work of all participating field research centers. As the WHO's archives document, all memoranda and correspondence between headquarters and participating countries, no matter how developed, were sent telegraphically. International communication had been established.

Standardizing Diagnostic Tools

By the late 1950s, experts at the WHO were already familiar with international processes of data collection, dissemination, and analysis. The global study of mental disorders still faced obstacles, however. The study required defining mental disorders as discrete diseases, each with its own etiology, manifestations, course, and prognosis. These disease profiles were essential to any consideration of the social, economic, or even cultural determinants of a mental disorder. The WHO's International Social Psychiatry Project thus sought to develop disease profiles so that classification within social groups could proceed from an examination of those already diagnosed with a given disease. The project required meticulous efforts and the kind of epidemiological knowledge at which the WHO excelled.

While a working group at the Mental Health Unit was trying to unify diagnostic criteria for mental disorders, another group was considering the sense in which a mental disorder can be said to exist in different parts of the world, posing many corollary questions. For example, do mental disorders differ in form or content? Are they comparable? This group also wanted to know whether reliable techniques were available for recording and classifying symptomatology. Initially, psychiatrists in Geneva had decided to study schizophrenia, agreeing that its primary features were the most obvious. Introduced in chapter 3, the renowned International Pilot Study of Schizophrenia (IPSS) laid the groundwork for the long-term objectives of the WHO's epidemiological program on mental health.

Like many other survey studies, the IPSS needed a standardized instrument. In modern times, the instrument is often a questionnaire consisting of technical terms familiar to researchers. In the case of the IPSS, the instrument was different. Scientists used the Present State Examination (PSE) schedule, a guide to structuring clinical interviews developed by John Wing at the Institute of Psychiatry. It was first developed in 1967 as a list of items that systematically covered all likely phenomena considered during the examination of a patient's present mental condition. It also indicated how those phenomena should be coded. With the PSE, the examiner does not merely record the patient's answers to questions on a schedule but instead scrutinizes the patient's psychopathological features and applies clear definitions of clinical terms. The PSE thus converts symptoms observed in the interviewee to language understood by research psychiatrists. The PSE contains approximately five hundred questions, or items, each probing for a specific symptom or psychological phenomenon, and the examiner must determine whether the patient has a given symptom. The questions appear

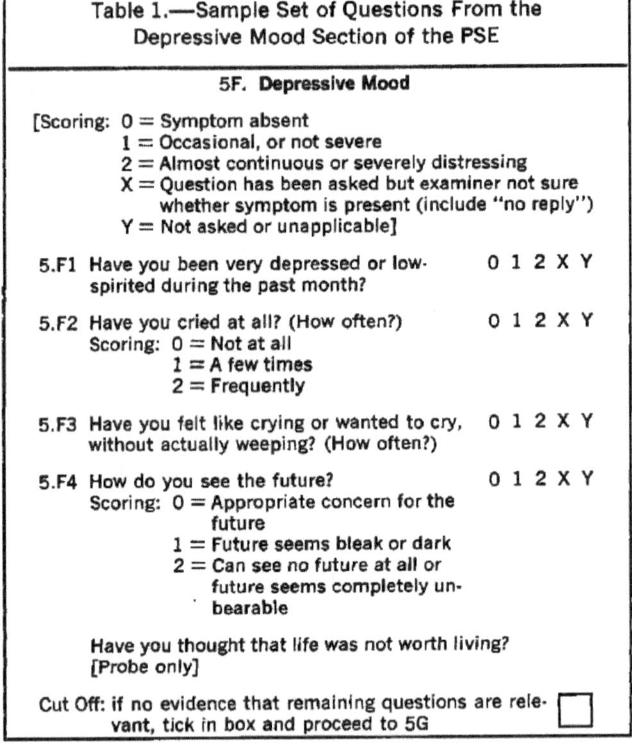

Table 1.—Sample Set of Questions From the Depressive Mood Section of the PSE

5F. Depressive Mood

[Scoring: 0 = Symptom absent
1 = Occasional, or not severe
2 = Almost continuous or severely distressing
X = Question has been asked but examiner not sure whether symptom is present (include "no reply")
Y = Not asked or unapplicable]

5.F1 Have you been very depressed or low-spirited during the past month? 0 1 2 X Y

5.F2 Have you cried at all? (How often?) 0 1 2 X Y
Scoring: 0 = Not at all
1 = A few times
2 = Frequently

5.F3 Have you felt like crying or wanted to cry, without actually weeping? (How often?) 0 1 2 X Y

5.F4 How do you see the future? 0 1 2 X Y
Scoring: 0 = Appropriate concern for the future
1 = Future seems bleak or dark
2 = Can see no future at all or future seems completely unbearable

Have you thought that life was not worth living? [Probe only]

Cut Off: if no evidence that remaining questions are relevant, tick in box and proceed to 5G ☐

Figure 5.1
Sample set of questions from the depressive mood section of the PSE.
Source: Richard E. Luria and Paul R. McHugh, "Reliability and Clinical Utility of the Wing Present State Examination," *Archives of General Psychiatry* 30, no. 6 (1974): 867.

in a sequence, with wording for initial probes, but the examiner may ask them in any manner that might induce the interviewee to express the designated symptom and must then judge whether a given symptom adhered to standard definitions.[16] To help collaborators in different field research centers understand and conduct interviews according to the PSE, WHO examiners thus also needed training.

The Mental Health Unit sought to ensure uniformity and reliability across interviews, but in developing interview questions, researchers encountered difficulty with translations into seven languages: Chinese, Czech, Danish, Hindi, Russian, Spanish, and Yoruba. To address the problem, the Mental Health Unit favored active participation by experienced, Geneva-based research scientists at the various FRCs.[17] Two doctors were sent from Geneva to each FRC to supervise local psychiatrists' use of the PSE, but they first went to London, where the PSE had been developed and inter-investigator reliability was tested, to view films of interviews with schizophrenic patients. The doctors then prepared an instruction manual for use before phase I of the IPSS (planned for April 1967).[18]

The politics and procedures of the WHO's mental health program imposed standardization. After selecting their FRCs, researchers began investigating the background conditions at all psychiatric centers involved, studying facilities, number of beds, staffing, and resources. Participating scientists standardized the observational methods that informed their judgments, thus corroborating what historians of science have deemed the construction of "objectivity."[19] The program's limited resources were equally distributed across FRCs, each of which was equipped with standardized equipment: two one-way screens, a calculator, a typewriter, a copier with supplies, a tape recorder, two air conditioners, a file cabinet, and a file drawer. To maximize uniformity across observations, one-way screens were limited in size to 100 cm × 50 cm. The project then established uniform methods for screening admitted patients and for collecting data on the numbers and types of psychiatric patients. Each patient had to be fifteen years or older, and "free of organic or physical diseases."[20] Even letters circulated to all the FRCs were presented in the same format. Apparently, scientists imagined a standard environment that could enable them to reach a shared objectivity in identifying mental symptoms.

Standardization aimed to minimize the influence of human variability, but its implementation required human authority. One of the letters to the FRCs from Tsung-yi Lin stated that "Scientists participating in the study will try to devise and to apply standard methods of identifying schizophrenics." They will attempt, the letter instructed, to "agree on standard ways to describe the psychological and behavioral characteristics of schizophrenic patients, and for determining the effect that cultural and social differences have on the course of the disease."[21] While the FRCs carried out diagnostic exercises, the WHO supplied supervisors and staff to ensure consistency in all elements of the study. As the study protocol concluded, the diagnostic exercises "contributed greatly to the elucidation of areas of agreement and disagreement in the diagnostic practices of different psychiatrists and make it possible to come closer to a mutual understanding."[22] Lin's persistence demanded conformity but also ensured the smooth progress of the research agenda.

Translation, Language, and Misunderstandings: Problems with the PSE

Controversies about standardization extended to the translation of diagnostic criteria and instruments. English and French were the WHO's official languages, but the language to be used in papers prepared for project seminars and diagnostic exercises was often debated, with those speaking Latin-derived languages, such as Portuguese, preferring French.[23] A precedent of sorts was established in 1957, when the World Psychiatric Association held its second meeting in Zurich and published its proceedings in both English and Interlingua, an international auxiliary language (IAL) based on European languages and designed to be scientific, natural, and practical.[24] This conference was the only one to employ that bilingual policy, however. The WHO's International Social Psychiatry Project had begun in London, where its leaders naturally employed English, and Tsung-yi Lin also favored English as the project's official language. Before the experts' first meeting on the classification of psychiatric diagnoses in October 1965, some potential participants had suggested that all meeting conversations be translated into other languages, but Lin, as project leader, did not think this step necessary. He proposed that during the conference, only English texts be prepared while the videotapes were shown.[25]

Translation of the PSE, however, posed challenges. Headquarters wanted to ensure that FRCs presented questions that were as uniform as possible. Expressions and examples were chosen carefully, and idiolects (individual speech habits) were avoided. Back-translation assessed the quality of translation and ensured equivalence in meaning; it was used during the first two phases of the program for descriptions of symptoms from all FRCs.[26] But the principal communication challenges were rooted in cross-cultural misunderstandings and differences in the basic concepts of psychiatric diseases across societies and cultures. For example, while translating the PSE schedule, experts found it impossible to translate the words "zombie," "automation," and "robot" because the terms were understood differently in various cultures that shared the same language. In the final report of the IPSS, those terms were better understood by "a middle-class European" than by other patients included in the study (table 5.1).[27]

Early opposition to the PSE came especially from the National Institute of Mental Health (NIMH) in Bethesda, Maryland. For example, the term "friend" used in the psychosocial history form mentioned social relationships in the context of evaluating social withdrawal, but the word had no clear definition and was thus difficult to translate.[28] Questions such as "Can God communicate with you?" were also disapproved, as they occupied a gray zone between faith and psychopathology.[29] Lyman Wynne of the NIMH refused to use the PSE screening forms designed at the WHO

Table 5.1
An example of back-translation for the PSE Schedule

Original description: "Does some other force than yourself make you do, feel or say things that you do not intend? As though you were an automaton, robot (zombie), marionette, puppet, without a will of your own?"

Back-translation of the second sentence from	
Spanish	Do you feel like an automaton, or a mechanical doll (living death, marionette, puppet)?
Yoruba	As if you were an image without your own will (fairies, image, and others)?
Danish	As if you were an automaton or a robot without a will of your own?
Hindi	As though you are an automatic instrument or a puppet which does not have its own will (zombie, marionette, puppet, other)?
Chinese	As though you were an automatic machine or a robot without a will of your own (some supernatural power that revives the corpse, marionette, puppet, others)?
Czech	As if you would be some automaton, robot-machines (a plaything, a doll)?

headquarters. In a communication with the project leader, he wrote, "We have felt that the screening forms coming from Geneva were in certain ways more impractical for use here than the forms that we had developed.... I think that the problem stems from the fact that each of the three groups involved in writing the forms, Geneva, London, and Bethesda, has a somewhat different experience and different outlook, as well as different facilities and problems."[30]

Lin suppressed opposition from Bethesda and elsewhere, but the comments from the NIMH became fiercer and longer, and the trans-Atlantic quarrel became a serious obstacle, even delaying the WHO's research schedule. For example, US psychiatrist Lyman Wynne (1923–2007), who was known for his research work in schizophrenia, noted that delays were expected because "we have put a lot of time into working on the forms and in thinking about the conceptualizations.... With the difficulties of transatlantic communication, and with the busy schedules that we all have in Geneva, Bethesda, and London, I am sure that there will be continuing problems in keeping each other up to date."[31]

Demands from NIMH included condensing interview instruments and seeking greater accuracy in translation. According to the Bethesda experts, expecting a huge document to be used, in its original form, "right away" in all FRCs was unrealistic.[32] Lin continued to suppress many objections, not only because he wanted the work to go on without much revision but also because his project's success depended on his own managerial charisma.

A Managerial Leader

Standardization was the most common way to pursue objectivity in scientific research. Ironically, however, to achieve standardization when the WHO's internal politics affected trust in the Mental Health Unit, a powerful individual was required as a troubleshooter to decide what was to be standardized and how to achieve it. Individuals who took the lead had to make sure that projects were carried out smoothly, without great objections. In a few recollections, Lin was described as an entrepreneurial individual who was not easy to approach. A careful listener and eloquent communicator, however, he mediated and coordinated among numerous comments and opinions. Many of his colleagues remembered his ability to quickly summarize complex research conducted by different researchers, integrating each researcher's expertise to further his own agenda.[33] After Lin left the WHO, Norman Sartorius, the head of the Mental Health Section, took Lin's post on the interregional team on the Epidemiology of Mental Disorders and continued the work of drafting *ICD-9*. He, too, was described as a bold and charismatic leader.[34] Those abilities were needed to transcend internal conflicts and to mobilize a vast organization. Under his leadership, IPSS and DOSMED were completed in 1973 and 1992, respectively. Because he was the one who completed these projects, Sartorius became the more celebrated leader of WHO's work in mental health.

The language skills of psychiatrists at the WHO headquarters and the FRCs were also a factor in overcoming obstacles. Almost all, including Sartorius, were bilingual or even trilingual, and at least fluent in English. These professionals accepted the validity of the cross-cultural and cross-language comparisons.[35] Sharing similar cultural experiences and objectives, they viewed the International Social Psychiatry Project's method of inquiry as valid and trustworthy. Local investigators at the FRCs, however, were often less convinced. For example, Erik Ströngren, from Aarhus, Denmark, commented on the report of the second Geneva meeting, saying "it could only give meaning to me, if not only the psychiatrists, but also [if] the patient were bilingual, which on the other hand, is not very probable."[36] Such disputes appeared in correspondence between headquarters and FRCs. Nonetheless, although the third and fourth phases of the International Social Psychiatry Project were delayed, the first two phases were completed in 1975, in time for *ICD-9*.

According to Lin, the "common interest" among experts and their esprit de corps made the program possible.[37] As with other WHO programs, however, hierarchical power played a part. For example, according to Chu-Chang Chen, director of the FRC in Taiwan, Lin chose Taiwan as an FRC for the International Social Psychiatry Project partly for personal reasons. Lin not only communicated easily with colleagues from his home country, but also, by choosing Taipei as an obligatory travel destination, he could visit his homeland during the years he was blacklisted by his government due to the political ideology he had developed abroad.[38] Lin's strength of personality was an asset in administering the project. Nevertheless, interpersonal factors hampered its smooth progress, and he left Geneva in 1969 because of private discord with the chief of the Mental Health Unit, Peter Baan. Two years later, Taiwan ceased to represent China in the WHO.[39]

The Promises of Technology

In the early 1960s, when recent scientific innovations during the Cold War had led to the space race and the threat of nuclear war, experts at the WHO turned to the promise of technology. Over time, scientists and their organizations had come to see technological neutrality as the freedom to acquire the most applicable measure to fulfill their needs in problem solving, developing infrastructure, and even commercializing research products. Nevertheless, toward the end of the twentieth century social scientists critiqued the *ICD*, one of the WHO's most important products, noting its political problems and uncertain technical underpinnings. Many saw the *ICD* as a mechanism for information processing that codified mistakes and obscured cultural variations; others saw it as a form of technology, bound by its limited data storage and processing.[40] As a part of the International Social Psychiatry Project, the WHO's Mental Health Unit laid the groundwork for *ICD-9*'s fifth chapter, which presented a classification of mental disorders. Much like the standardization of interview tools, classification raised questions that challenged the neutrality of knowledge making. It is irrefutable, however, that standardization and classification were driving forces for the project.

Videotaping

To make symptoms of mental illness measurable, they first had to be visualized. During the interwar period, medicine had incorporated technologies for documentation in hospital records, which included evaluations of symptoms, decisions on treatments, and monitoring disease progression. By the mid-twentieth century, motion picture technology had transformed narrative, allowing nature to be presented through time-lapse images rather than still forms. Zoologists used video cameras to capture images of wildlife, rendering the subtleties of the wilderness visible. Cell biologists used cinematography to capture the action of cells.[41] Technologies that shaped scientific knowledge thus readily included the new discipline of psychiatry and eventually its new diagnostic criteria for mental disorders.

Psychiatrists' use of imaging technologies has had a long history. Scientists might hesitate to claim to have accurate pictures of pathological minds, but they believed cameras could help them witness the truth and have never been reluctant to develop diagnostic measures with up-to-date imaging technology. Photography, for example, was adopted as a tool for observation, an instrument for archiving, and a medium for the delivery of knowledge. In the 1850s, Hugh W. Diamond (1809–1886) had used calotypes to capture the facial expressions of individuals who suffered from mental disturbances. His work was the origin of psychiatric photography.[42] According to Diamond, "Photography gives permanence to these remarkable cases, which are types of classes, and makes them observable not only now but forever, and it presents also a perfect and faithful record."[43] Diamond even became one of the first psychiatrists to employ visual technology for developing diagnoses. In Britain, his reputation became greater in the field of photography than in psychiatry. Later, Jean-Martin Charcot (1825–1893), a neurologist as well as keeper of the museum in Salpêtrière Hospital in Paris, famously described types of hysteria with the aid of photography.[44] Beyond these pioneers, psychiatric photography was employed in multiple contexts and for various purposes. Photographs illustrated trends in diagnosis and also served to stereotype groups, thus contributing to racial science and colonialism. For example, Edward Margetts (1920–2004), a Canadian psychiatrist who served as an expert consultant for the WHO, developed his interest in using photography to document patients' symptoms while he worked in western Kenya during the 1950s.[45] The method enabled him to document several conventional treatments of mental disorders there and to frame his theory, which resembled the racial stereotype of Carothers's "African mind" (see chapter 2).

In the second half of the twentieth century, visual technology evolved from the capacity to capture still images to capturing moving ones. Videotaping developed in tandem with new psychological theories that informed the design of the WHO's diagnostic exercises. Video technology inspired the renowned psychiatrist John Bowlby to tape the experiences of children who had been separated from their parents in wartime. In postwar Britain, the Children's Department of the County Borough of Croydon ran a series of programs to analyze possible causes of family failure and to devise preventive strategies.[46] A central concern was the care of children whose mothers were unmarried, divorced, or widowed. Not long after this program ran, Bowlby spoke at a WHO planning conference on the psychological development of children: "My particular interest is in the effects on personality development of separation from the mother in the first three to four years of life," he explained. "This situation, with particular reference to the reactions of a very acute and emotional nature which follow it, gives the best opportunity to study the connection between real experience and later personality deviations."[47] To prove the evidence of these children's experiences, he relied on film records.

In April 1948, at the third session of the Social Commission of the United Nations, delegates decided to initiate a study of homeless children, and in 1950, Bowlby took leave from the Tavistock Clinic to take an appointment at the WHO, leading a project on this topic initiated by the Sir Halley Stewart Trust. Bowlby's project partner, James Robertson (1911–1988), a psychiatric social worker and psychoanalyst, recognized the potential of the cine-camera to strengthen the presentation of human behavior and reveal social problems to an audience. In 1948, at the Central Middlesex Hospital in London, he joined Bowlby's project to observe and film children separated from their parents. Robertson's work demonstrated the power of film. In his first film, the 1951 *A Two-Year-Old Goes to Hospital,* he used a small hand-held camera to capture the severe emotional stress that two-year-old Laura displayed during an eight-day hospital stay, despite the thorough care of hospital staff. His film became evidence of children's emotional needs when separated from their parents, especially their mothers.

For Robertson, the narrative of video and film was a means to approximate the truth. In an article detailing the process, he elaborated: "The aim in filming a social situation for the purpose of discussion is to capture actuality with a minimum of distortion. Audiences can then match what they are shown against their own experience and beliefs." What is shown, Robertson asserted, must be "authentic and not reconstructed."[48] Recognizing that the new technology could cause anxiety in his subjects, Robertson took care in preparation, arranging the setting to document human emotions with minimum invasion. Although *A Two-Year-Old Goes to Hospital* looked like a film that was produced off the cuff, its production took the crew fifteen months of planning, with Robertson anticipating unexpected circumstances, including lighting changes, weather conditions, and human behavior that might compromise the control of conditions during filming. For example, in an 11-by-9-foot cubicle with a cot, bed, locker, and chair, setting up a tripod was impractical, so a skillful camera operator familiar with the environment captured all activities.

Robertson's film contributed to Bowlby's efforts to popularize the view that prolonged parental deprivation caused mental health problems in children. Bowlby was then a member of the Expert Committee in the WHO's Mental Health Unit. Consistent with the WHO's project on maternal care, his concern was etiology. Bowlby's work responded to the Social Commission's call to study "children who are orphaned or separated from their families for other reasons and need care in foster homes, institutions or other types of group care."[49] Unlike the Social Commission's report, which was confined to homeless children in their native countries, Bowlby's work went further to include refugees from wars and other disasters.[50]

The Mental Health Expert Committee also participated in the study of juvenile delinquency.[51] Expert views of juvenile delinquency varied, but many supported the UN's vision for preventing crime and treating offenders. Bowlby's theory of parent-child separation, however, corresponded with Director-General Brock Chisholm's emphasis on the value and purpose of the family, and it fit other WHO projects related to maternal care. Bowlby's project ultimately became one of the WHO's first monographs, *Maternal Care and Mental Health*, published in 1951, which addressed a range of adverse effects caused in children by maternal deprivation before the rise of feminism focused attention on women's well-being. The monograph became the major source of Bowlby's renowned attachment theory.

Clearly, Robertson and Bowlby were not the only ones who saw the feasibility of using visual technology in mental health works. Thomas L. Pilkington, the chairman of the executive board and the film consultant at the World Federation of Mental Health, was enthusiastic about establishing in Geneva an international audiovisual center concerned with mental health. Realizing the educative and therapeutic functions of films, the federation persistently worked during its first decade on the "World Catalogue of Mental Health Films."[52] For Pilkington himself, film was powerful not only because it promoted the importance of mental health to the general public, but also because it was a convenient means to spread information about new techniques and methods of care. He and others assumed, for example, that the development of simple audiovisual aids—film, radio, television, and tape recorders—was useful for educational purposes in schools where medical resources were lacking, such as in Africa.[53]

Film could indeed be used for medical instruction. More important, it was the only medium in which a real-life visual and sound representation could be made and preserved. Because of its unique nature, film was eventually used to compare psychiatric symptomology in different cultural patterns in the WHO's International Social Psychiatry Project. In Pilkington's words, "[films] can transmit new thinking in mental health treatment and rehabilitation, they can contrast etiology and psychiatric stresses, they can present incidence and contrast epidemiology in a realistic way."[54]

The International Social Psychiatry Project employed the same careful techniques in videography that had guided the scientific work and plans discussed above. The project not only encouraged patients to describe their symptoms on camera but also ensured standard conditions for filming. As the medical officer of the Mental Health Unit, Tsung-yi Lin recollected that upon his first visit to the United States, in 1950, he had been dazzled by the video-recording technology at Chicago's Museum of Science and Industry, an excitement chronicled later in his personal memoir.[55] However, the first generation of videotape machines were "formidable" as they were bulky, noisy, and usually overheated.[56] At the WHO, experts had similarly placed their hope and trust in this new technology. In London, before the inauguration of the IPSS, the US/UK team at the Institute of Psychiatry had developed a mobile videotape studio that was already far more user-friendly.[57] Videotaped interviews were shown to American and British psychiatrists, who noted "striking differences" in diagnoses in their two countries but, with a video record, could argue that dissimilar diagnostic criteria were the main cause of the differences.[58]

The WHO thus sought to avoid research bias by strictly regulating investigators' subjective visual experiences. Equipment used in the diagnostic exercises for the first phase of the International Social Psychiatry Project was selected to ensure that observations of patients in different environments were consistently collected. The apparatus included a movie projector that ran 16-mm film at a speed of 24 fps and standard videotape reels, 2,400 feet long, with a diameter of 14 inches. All filmed interviews were transcribed, proofread, and typed onto a ditto master.[59] For translations, experts discussed dubbing tapes in local languages and establishing an audio-video laboratory. The Institute of Psychiatry in London expressed great interest in this idea, and to this end, it sought a film company.[60]

Data Management Technology

During the early development of computing technology, analysts compared the function and calculating capacity of computers with that of human brains. During World War II, it was the question, "Can machines think?" that stimulated the development of computing technologies.[61] At Bletchley Park, for example, Alan Turing's calculating machine assisted the Allies in decoding Enigma, the apparatus used by Nazi Germany for communication. At the same institution, technology was also developed to research Nazi communications and persuasion. Toward the end of World War II, scientists began to develop an obsession with cybernetics. It was in a mental health hospital that the first cybernetic machine was invented, gaining worldwide attention. Ross Ashby (1903–1972), the chief of research at Barnwood House, a private mental health hospital in Gloucester, England, and a major in the Royal Army Medical Corps, was inspired by the mentally ill patients with whom he worked. In 1949, he told *Time* magazine that his machine, the Homeostat, was "the closest thing to a synthetic human brain so far designed by man."[62] In addition, historians have gradually unearthed unethical research by the US psychologist Carl Hovland (1912–1961) and Canadian psychiatrist Ewen Cameron, who used new technology to understand and potentially affect the enemy's mental state. Their research continued into the Cold War period, with investigations of technological means to alter the human mind, which placed Cameron under suspicion after his involvement in the CIA's MK-Ultra "brain-washing" project.[63] Despite critiques from historians of science, this research pioneered psychiatry's interest in technology to study human learning and cognitive processes.[64] Later, for example, Hovland developed a computer simulation of human thought processing, applying a new mathematical theory to explain the way human brains form new concepts.

After World War II, the medical sciences engaged in an active knowledge exchange with technological disciplines. Renowned US neurophysiologist and cybernetician Warren McCulloch (1898–1969), invited to address the American Institute of Electrical Engineers in 1949, asserted, "the notion of ultimate units has been applied to the communications field and has opened the way to important advances in the design of calculating machines and to a better understanding of the working of our brains."[65] His remark implied that brain scientists heavily relied on computing technology, not only for data storage but also for processing and interpretation. Evidence also shows that, after World War II, the United States military employed cybernetics in a way that enhanced psychiatry's exercise of power. For example, under Dwight Eisenhower's presidency, the RAND Corporation used computers to establish mathematical models and to create analyzable scenarios, and the government sponsored follow-up psychological tests among veterans to explore psychological warfare.[66]

With the slow development of software programs during the first decade of the postwar period, however, the gap remained wide between such high hopes to precisely capture the absolute mental symptoms and their realization. Not until 1960 did the US surgeon general approve the Computation and Data Processing Branch in the Division of Research Services at the National Institutes of Health, in Bethesda, Maryland. Then, in April 1964, the Division of Computer Research and Technology was established. Technologies for data management also evolved over the course of the International Social Psychiatry Project. In 1965, a conference was organized to discuss the complementary roles computers might play in mental health, electronic clinical record systems, and patient management.[67] By then, computers could generate automated patient questionnaires and program languages, such as the Massachusetts General Hospital Utility Multi-programming System, or MUMPS, which could manage a database of patient records.[68] Moreover, in Bethesda, the NIH became the only mega-institution fully installed with a time-sharing computer developed by IBM. It proved useful for the more than three thousand scientists at the NIH's forty-eight-building complex.[69]

At the beginning of the International Pilot Study of Schizophrenia, the speed of data processing was so slow that FRCs were unable to carry out the task and instead sent data on symptoms to the WHO headquarters, which then sent them for further processing to London or Bethesda. Toward the end of 1965, the maintenance of the Camberwell register, in London, for example, became too cumbersome for punch cards, and in 1966, the database was transferred to magnetic tapes on the London University Atlas Computer, which two private companies, Ferranti and Plessey, had jointly developed with the University of Manchester. When commissioned, it was considered the world's speediest supercomputer.[70] London University's Atlas Computer belonged to the second generation. It was smaller, with only 16,000 words of core storage, eight Ampex tape decks, four paper tape readers, three punches, two card readers, one card punch, and two Anelex printers. With this equipment, a piecemeal system for updating the register tapes was developed, allowing analysis of data from different hospitals. Much later, a series of major analysis programs aimed to produce regular and reliable yearly statistics that were applied in the Camberwell register.[71]

Computing Software

With developments in hardware, software was critical, too. Toward the end of the 1960s, the proliferation of new software resulted in the replacement of labor-intensive record keeping and processing.[72] Before the advent of commercial software in the late 1960s, scientists had written instructions directing computers to perform specific tasks, and yet computers could now compile and categorize large sets of data.[73] To solve the complex problem of analysis, British psychiatrist John Wing wrote CATEGO, a software program that categorized psychopathological descriptions of symptoms, leading him to operationalize the classification of mental disorders. Having developed the PSE interview instrument for data collection,[74] Wing had masterminded a system for analysis. The CATEGO classification could work with the *ICD* system, which was then under revision. It could also identify cases deemed "double diagnoses," or instances of "comorbidity." Tsung-yi Lin praised the computer as being "different from clinicians' diagnoses.... It works for us carefully and objectively. Therefore, the exactness, trustworthiness, fixity, and integrity could be ensured. And it is also neutral without partiality."[75]

US clinicians attempted to use *DSM-II* in computer diagnostic systems in the 1960s, but their efforts failed not only because of the software but also because of the classification system.[76] *DSM-II* was neither verifiable among varying diagnostic approaches nor reliable, due to its weak and ambiguous nomenclature.[77] In Geneva, however, the Mental Health Unit used software to verify diagnoses. During IPSS diagnostic exercises, 1,202 sets of case records and PSE schedules were collected and stored, and CATEGO then narrowed the symptoms into categories in ten stages.[78] For example, in the first stage, the symptom "delusions of control" comprised six items, each of which could be scored zero, one, or two, so that, if all items were rated two, the overall score would be twelve. If any one item was fully present or if any two were partially present, the computer was instructed to record the symptom as present. If only one item was present, the rating was one, and if all items were rated zero, the symptom was considered absent.

CATEGO's second stage combined the symptoms to form thirty-five syndromes. For example, the first syndrome consisted of five symptoms that Kurt Schneider (1887–1967), in 1938, first considered characteristic of schizophrenia: auditory hallucinations, thought broadcast, thought insertion, thought withdrawal, and delusional perception. These symptoms, known as "first rank symptoms," are nowadays still believed by many practicing psychiatrists to be the essential features of schizophrenia. The CATEGO program then instructed the computer to print out the syndromes present, together with their degrees of certainty and scores. These data constituted the basic descriptive material for disease classification. In subsequent stages, the program incorporated roles for combing through thirty-five syndromes to allocate to each patient only a few descriptive categories, based on the symptoms rated in the PSE.

Bewilderment about Technology

Occasionally, experts found new technology bewildering, mostly because they distrusted the hermeneutic capacity of artificial intelligence to describe a person's mental status. Such unease appeared irregularly among psychiatrists and other health professionals. Yet technology became central to the development of psychiatry over the course of the 1960s, a decade of cultural and political change. For example, although *A Two-Year-Old Goes to Hospital* upset many hospital staff, who felt punished despite their good deeds, it became an influential educational film that played a critical role in promoting greater understanding of hospitalized children and their need for parental visits and play. Moreover, over the century-long history of psychiatry, whether or not mental suffering could be visualized under the so-called neurological gaze of film technology was still the subject of heated debate.[79]

Technology has always been a source of anxiety as well as hope, obsession, and dependence. During the closing session of the fourth WHO classification seminar in 1968, Dr L. Angyal, from Hungary, questioned the use of film as a demonstration method. In his view, the "human brain does not work like a calculating machine," and he suggested developing "fresh elaboration" and "the enlarging of the symptoms." Rather than refining evaluation techniques, he hoped for "highly developed electronic computer techniques" that would achieve a "five-digit subdivision" that would expand the *ICD*'s three-digit system.[80] His call controverted the *ICD* task force's initial effort to avoid a difficult and complex system. And ironically, such a view has been adopted by health insurance companies. The technology, however, now had an established path.

Fallacies of Neutrality

To classify is human, claim sociologists of scientific knowledge. This statement presents two implications.[81] One is that classification is a natural human behavior, while the other suggests that any glossary produced might reflect the producers' value judgments and worldview, and thus classification can be arbitrary. When the International Social Psychiatry Project in Psychiatric Epidemiology and Social Psychiatry sought to standardize metrics to measure symptoms of mental illness, the project traded official local statistics for a system of international comparison, which the United Nations and its specialized agencies deemed a pressing need. The health and illness data that the WHO compiled reflected the priorities of the UN and other specialized agencies to standardize, coordinate, and compile sets of international data. The process, however, translated disparate cultures and so shaped not only the character of the institution but also the content of the scientific claims.[82] The social psychiatry project thus established a method of knowing.

Despite some scientists' ambivalence, technology was central to the WHO's social psychiatry project. Technology shaped the trajectory of knowledge, as scientists developed new technologies to surpass the limitations they faced. Experts across scientific disciplines identified and built upon technological artifacts that could operate as "boundary objects," guiding and informing practitioners from different disciplines as they coordinated their work.[83] Although technology was important, it was still a boundary object that served human imagination about what technology could do. The WHO's technology was "both plastic enough to adapt to local needs and the constraints of the several parties employing them, yet robust enough to maintain a common identity across sites."[84] Not all scientists understood the technology. For example, the first project coordinator, Tsung-yi Lin, recalled his own difficulty in understanding the complex algorithm of a hierarchical clustering technique developed by J. J. McKeon, in addition to CATEGO analysis, which he was more familiar with.[85] Besides, all collected data were sent for processing at the National Institutes of Health in Bethesda, as the computing system was also unknown in Geneva and London. Yet technology reflected the shared wishful thinking that computers could undertake tasks that were beyond the capabilities of human computation. Technology was employed by project planners, statisticians, and collaborating clinicians, all of whom believed it critical in achieving their common goals. At that time, however, scientists were not yet able to foresee the risk of human beings becoming numbers extrapolated from their identities, personalities, and cultures.

At the WHO, project participants acted on their consensus view of world citizenship, an idea that might be termed a boundary concept.[86] Perhaps world citizenship was most fully understood only by Brock Chisholm, but it provided a loose and flexible goal that gave the project meaning. Early on, the WHO's scientists had agreed to imagine "universal criteria of mental disorders." The technology employed in the WHO's International Social Psychiatry Projects was multifold, but it was never neutral. The outcome of the research achieved a certain degree of objectivity, but technology was also accused of "flattening" science by imposing rigid criteria, too inflexible to encompass a wider range or nuance in disease classification. For instance, criticized by Assen Jablensky, a top scholar in psychiatric classification, the rigidity of nosology resulted in clinician's reluctance to separate some apparent mental disorders, such as schizophrenia and affective disorders that share similar symptoms, and further find effective solutions to classify non-pathological forms of cognitive and emotional deviations.[87]

The WHO is a unique institution. After seven decades, it still reflects the quasi-utopian scientific internationalism of the immediate post-World War II period, despite critiques of its bureaucracy and North-South developmentalism. In mobilizing such a large unit as the Mental Health Unit and its collaborators to conduct a manageable project, the organization depended on the people who established its methods for standardization. Internally, leading individuals needed to be competent enough to deal with the complex administrative workload. Externally, they had to overcome the restrictions of their own state citizenship and the limitations imposed by international relations. Reacting to the devastation of war and led by the ideal of worldwide collaboration, scientists participated in the manufacture of a "world standard." By fulfilling the promise of universality, however, the project sacrificed a more decentralized, democratic mode of knowledge production in which all participants might share equally as contributors and beneficiaries.

As Jacques Derrida noted, the archive itself reflects violence.[88] Archiving things destroys alternative presentations in different temporal and spatial contexts. Videography at the WHO exemplified such violence. It captured, in detail, the symptoms of mental disorders, but only those of patients recruited in hospitals available to the nine FRCs. Missing, for example, are sites without psychiatric services. Scientists wrote software to analyze the symptoms of mental disorders they collected through videos, and they aspired to develop more commanding machines to add nuance to their categorization of mental symptoms. But in their zeal to represent the world with standardized methods, they also enacted Derrida's archival fallacy. In the years to come, peoples' psychic worlds and their moral understanding of normality and insanity would be mediated by technologies that were originally assumed to be impersonal and unbiased. Standardization thus reflected both the competence and the inadequacy of the scientists who carried out the WHO's Social Psychiatric Project.

6 Discontent

Experts at the WHO reached a consensus when they resolved to study the universal profiles of mental disorders and, subsequently, to classify them. In Geneva, the spirit of "world citizenship" not only pervaded the atmosphere but also informed the project. Psychiatrists recruited to the International Social Psychiatry Project envisioned an attainable method through which they could meet their goals. Their design for international collaboration in science mirrored the zeitgeist of the WHO. Yet real-life conditions—institutional bureaucracy, international relations during the Cold War, dependence on technology, and changing methodology—hindered a truly democratic process for producing scientific knowledge. After a honeymoon period, new theories and approaches arose again to critique a universal, totalizing, and metrical view of mental disorders.

Discontent grew with the WHO's work. Scarce funding, inadequate resources, and a shortage of manpower compared with that of the agency's infectious disease programs overshadowed the WHO's achievement in social psychiatry in the 1970s. Functioning under layers of difficulties, it developed its own model of knowledge production, which regrettably resembled manufacturing systems that subcontract segments of their process. The WHO espoused collaboration with developing countries, but its first large-scale mental health research project was not as decentralized and democratic as its experts claimed. The experts viewed health as an economic problem, and so the WHO's original objective was to improve health in developing countries by boosting their economies. Economic life did indeed improve to varying degrees, especially in Asia, and health, too, became substantially better. One factor facilitating this economic development was the export processing model of production in which developing countries conformed to specifications designed by the WHO.

Instead of manufacturing tangible products, the model employed by the WHO produced scientific knowledge through a decentralized organizational structure, a mechanism for outsourcing, and a metrical approach to classifying disease. But did the International Social Psychiatry Project meet the essence of world citizenship? Were its profiles of mental disorders sufficiently expanded worldwide? Was the newly established disease classification system as applicable as expected? Along with advancing the methods and content of psychiatric epidemiology, the scrutiny and characterization of mental disorders did, surely, improve. Today, revision of the *ICD* continues, and the system appears to be increasing its reach and expanding its application globally.

Internally Contested Methods

In the early 1970s, the International Pilot Study of Schizophrenia and the revision of mental disorders classified in *ICD-9* were the two global achievements of the WHO's International Social Psychiatry Project. The new disease classification system provided a gold standard, more encompassing than its predecessors, and it soon became beneficial for global mental health research. By the time IPSS ended, the Mental Health Unit had expanded to become a division under Norman Sartorius's leadership. The study also established the foundation for international psychiatric epidemiology. Its follow-up study, Determinants of Outcome of Severe Mental Disorders (DOSMED), established the lifetime prevalence of schizophrenia at approximately one to two percent of the entire human population. DOSMED provided strong evidence for the notion that schizophrenic illnesses occur with comparable frequency across all population groups, a view of disease prevalence that psychiatrists everywhere have come to consider valid.[1] The study revealed superior disease outcomes for individuals suffering from schizophrenia in developing countries. It has also become one of the most extensively cited research reports to support a variety of mental health plans in these countries.

Yet criticisms also began to emerge over the effectiveness of the WHO's research outcomes. Some researchers still saw schizophrenia as heterogeneous. For example, Cambridge University Professor Martin Roth (1917–2006) and his long-term psychologist collaborator H. McClelland stressed the need to consider a broader picture of schizophreniform syndromes. They thought the IPSS only revealed the nuclear criteria of the disorder, ignoring the fact that there were still individuals and populations who suffered from atypical but related symptoms.[2] There were fiercer critics, too, such as Alex Cohen, an eminent anthropologist at the London School of Hygiene and Tropical Medicine. Reviewing twenty-three longitudinal studies on schizophrenia outcomes in eleven lower- and middle-income countries and applying a consistent review method, Cohen and his colleagues concluded that the clinical outcomes, patterns of disease course, and disability and social outcomes of the disease necessitated further validation.[3] Commenting on the DOSMED study, these analysts showed that patients suffering from schizophrenia do not necessarily exhibit its expected outcomes. Rather, biomedical treatment, disability and social functioning, marriage and employment status, the role of families, and mortality and suicide vary across countries. This variability led Cohen and his colleagues to consider the heterogeneity of mental disorders across cultures to be the result of the social indicators they had identified. Their challenge rendered the DOSMED controversial. The WHO's research no longer produced reliable scientific axioms without controversies.

The IPSS's conclusion was, in fact, conservative. With nine countries participating, the study made no claims to universally valid diagnostic criteria for schizophrenia. Instead, it proved only the possibility of conducting a reliable cross-cultural study of the disease. Looking back at the research process, voices both inside and outside the WHO questioned the organization's lofty ambitions. Many of these early concerns prefigured today's heated debates in the field of global mental health. For example, when accepting Tsung-yi Lin's invitation to participate in the second phase of the program, Ernest Gruenberg, affiliated with the Milbank Memorial Fund, a project patron, articulated fundamental problems with disease classification: "First, the entire concept of starting with a single disorder on a small scale is acceptable," he noted, "but differences within one country or area are extremely difficult to quantify and are even more so in international contexts. Several cities have marked internal variations in sociocultural environments yet differences are difficult to objectify."[4] The project was also criticized for posing too many broad questions for a study with a limited timeline.[5]

The history of the WHO has included other projects begun with ample ambition but eventually narrowed in scale. In the International Social

Psychiatry Project, however, popular trends in psychiatry had to be sacrificed to satisfy the majority. One was the diagnostic tradition derived from Freudian psychopathology. Another was inclusion of psychotic reactive or psychogenic depressions, in which predominantly confusional (or hysterical) symptoms were difficult to integrate into the system.[6] These conditions were thus classified as manic-depressive psychosis or neuroses. Hans Strotzka (1917–1994), a Viennese psychiatrist, wrote to Lin commenting that "in the plans for the future meeting is no mention of 'neuroses and psychogenic reactions' which are the most common psychiatric disorders within a population and which need to be clarified most urgently."[7] Lorna Wing, a "consumer of ICD" and wife of John Wing, celebrated later for her research on Asperger syndrome, also commented on the validity of such a nosological system. According to her studies at Camberwell in the 1970s, more than 24 percent of psychiatric patients had underlying or precipitating causes of mental illness, and she criticized the *ICD* for its overreliance on phenomenology rather than psychopathology.[8]

Statisticians hired by the WHO expressed other concerns. They noted the language gap between scientists at the Geneva headquarters and clinicians in the field research centers. For example, London-trained health statistician Eileen Brooke (1905–1989) reported during the WHO project's very early stage that "classifications in the ICD were far from satisfied with the way the ICD had been working." She pointed out discord between the terms frequently used by psychiatrists who supplied data and the terms that described *ICD* categories. In addition, she raised concern that statistical data on patient registration were collected only from inpatients in mental health hospitals: "The material does not include data from psychiatric departments and observation wards of general hospitals, but they cater for [sic] only a very small proportion of the psychiatric patients."[9] Interestingly, in project seminars at WHO headquarters, Brooke was often the only woman at the roundtable with the male psychiatrists. Her comment became one of the rare contributions that redressed gender inequality in the masculine and chauvinistic culture of the WHO. Reflecting on the difficulty of collaboration between psychiatrists and statisticians, she said, "there is a problem in bringing about effective co-operation between these two specialists. One difficulty is due to differences in training. The statistician is taught to analyze, to take a large mass of data and divide it up into small groups. The clinician, on the other hand, is trained to synthesize, to take a variety of signs, messages and measurements, and weld them, for instance, into a diagnosis."[10] Even though her voice was rarely heard in this world of male physicians, she continued to work on the improvement of long-term healthcare information systems as a medical statistician.

Echoing Brooke's concern, John Wing suggested that the WHO incorporate the Camberwell patient register system that the Wings were developing. The database of the Camberwell register included patients who had undergone psychiatric services in any form, not just inpatients. Based on the Camberwell data, John and Lorna Wing had conducted a wide range of epidemiological surveys. One focused on psychotherapy, the most prevalent treatment method employed by psychiatrists, which was relevant for planning local psychotherapy services. The Wings first established the number of people in the register who had received psychotherapy, and with this information, they estimated the number of patients who had received outpatient treatment and who had been referred for psychotherapy. They found that the number of patients in the Camberwell register receiving outpatient treatment was twice that of other areas in southeast England and that the number of patients referred for psychotherapy was three times higher. The data further pointed to patients suffering from severe levels of mental illness in areas where psychiatric services were relatively plentiful. This positive correlation between accessibility of mental health services and the prevalence of mental disorders implied a causal relationship.

With this surprising outcome, halfway through the WHO's project, the Wings had warned that their research had a common limitation; as they noted, "one cannot draw clinical conclusions from purely statistical trends or differences.... The fact that more patients could have been referred for psychotherapy does not mean that more should have been."[11] Their research thus illustrated the symbiotic relationship between diagnostic tools and actual diseases. By implication, does the lack of satisfactory diagnostic language in a specific geographical area mean that mental health problems do not exist there? This early concern to some degree reflected criticisms later made by a number of scholars, stating that the IPSS did not reflect a uniformity of disease experience cross-culturally, especially outside of hospitals.[12] Currently, researchers attempt to answer this question through the refinement of epidemiology studies. Researchers now recruit patients not only from institutions but also through other catchment mechanisms in the area under investigation.

With the first two phases that the WHO's International Social Psychiatry Project initiated simultaneously, work on disease classification continued as disease profile research was developed. While the IPSS was in process, the WHO headquarters produced a glossary of definitions, collaboratively formulated by the investigators, to disambiguate the terms used in the study. The program was already at the end of its second year when the glossary appeared,[13] and it provoked disputes from different parts of the world. For example, from the National Institute of Mental Health in Bethesda, Maryland, John Strauss, who later became famous for challenging the disease entity concept of schizophrenia, argued for abandoning certain terms that could perpetuate ambiguity, as they were used differently by people from different backgrounds.[14] Investigators ultimately settled on operational definitions,[15] but at first, with both ad hoc and glossary definitions of symptoms, psychiatrists could advance their provisional work, leaving corrections and revisions for the future.

Not all participants complied strictly with the project's regulations. Some local scientists modified research methods to satisfy expectations at headquarters. This further explains participating scientists' eagerness to produce satisfactory data in an international scientific project. In Taiwan, for example, investigators Chu-Chang Chen and Ming-Tse Tsuang, who were both Lin's students, altered the study protocol formulated by WHO by interviewing patients consecutively rather than concurrently—that is, each patient was interviewed twice, once by each observer[16]—a protocol that minimized the use of ambiguous terms through expedient mutual agreement. As IPSS research proceeded, however, scientists observed that schizophrenic patients in the FRCs in Taipei and Cali generally showed values near the mean documented in Geneva.[17] In the case of Taiwan, this could be because participating psychiatrists in Taipei had a close relationship with Lin, first director of the IPSS.

Beyond Category Fallacies

One legacy of the International Social Psychiatry Project was the international classification of mental disorders. But the new classification of mental disorders did not seem to sufficiently account for the content of people's mental suffering. Interestingly, so-called culture-bound syndromes, including those reported in Lin's observations, were not included in the WHO research outcomes in *ICD-9*, published in 1975. One possible reason was that the identification of syndromes was proceeding worldwide; another reason could have been the WHO's ideology of world citizenship and its short-lived vision of an international scientific utopia. At the structural level, the World Federation for Mental Health—the organization established to advise the WHO's mental health cultural agenda—was gradually marginalized in the field of international social psychiatry. In the classification of diseases, culture as a determinant of psychopathology was held in abeyance until the next revision of the *ICD*. Culture-bound syndromes were endorsed by the World Health Assembly in 1990 and were officially adopted by the WHO's member countries in 1994, referred to as culture-specific disorders.[18] *ICD-10* thus corroborated the argument of epidemiologist and anthropologist Robert Hahn (1945–) that all diseases are culture-bound.[19] In the mid-1950s, however, the *ICD* was still bound to the optimistic notion of scientific internationalism and the organizational culture that supported it.

Problems related to the ideal of world citizenship thus emerged after IPSS, DOSMED, and the revision of *ICD-9* had concluded, when disease classification and diagnostic criteria were applied locally. Nonetheless, in the 1960s and 1970s, the WHO's experts analyzed diseases that were observed differently around the world. Some drew from the legacy of colonial racial science; others reflected emerging national identities amid decolonization. For example, some still deemed Africans to be genetically and culturally distinct, an assumption linked with the colonial racism evident in J. C. Carothers's writings and based principally on notions of an African biological constitution.[20] Experts in psychiatric epidemiology also criticized the WHO's classification of mental disorders for failing to account for cross-national manifestations of mental suffering, and eventually the field ceased to identify the occurrences of mental disorders quantitatively. Instead, to provide bases for intervention, researchers explored possible genetic, environmental, class, and cultural determinants. Consensus on the standardization of statistical systems for health in racial or ethnic populations was not attained until the 1990s, when ethnic health attracted attention in the United States.[21] From the 1970s onward, however, several novel approaches, embraced mostly by anthropologists who had conducted fieldwork, emphasized culture in the global study of mental disorders.

One of the most notable adherents of the view that some mental disorders are culturally mediated was Arthur Kleinman (1941–), a Harvard-based psychiatrist-anthropologist, who first studied tuberculosis in Taiwan in the 1970s and then further developed his famous research on depression and neurasthenia in China. As the first American psychiatrist who entered China behind the Iron Curtain, he contended that the standard method for cross-cultural psychiatry created categorical fallacies.[22] Kleinman ferociously criticized the neglect of greater China in the WHO's development of a disease classification system.[23] In fieldwork in Taiwan and China, he had found social suffering embedded in somatoform disorders that manifest themselves in specific social and political contexts. Moreover, he found, Chinese people used the more socially acceptable term *shenjing shuairuo* [neurasthenia] that had long existed in China rather than "depression," even though they referred to the same condition.[24] As Sing Lee, a student of Kleinman from Hong Kong, further noted, neurasthenia in China appeared in the post-Mao era as a product of multiple interests entrenched in complex historical, social, political, and economic processes. The "open door policy, the hegemony of *DSM* discourse, the depoliticization of experience, and the transnational commercialization of suffering" all contributed to the creation of such "new-found" disease categories.[25]

The WHO disputed Kleinman's critique, but the rediscovery of neurasthenia in China indicated a fundamental problem.[26] Designating Taiwan as the representative of China in the WHO's early years had generated inadequate samples of the population known as Chinese. This matter, however, went unexplored until the 1980s, when transcultural psychiatry became another pivotal chapter in the development of modern psychiatry. In the mid-1970s, diagnostic criteria were still presumed to be international standards, although only schizophrenia had been validated with cross-cultural epidemiological evidence, and the WHO had no plans for pilot studies to replicate its methods to look at other mental disorders. From the mid-1970s to the 2000s, the WHO gradually estimated the burden of mental disorders based on literature reviews and on limited and isolated studies in different countries. It further claimed that mental disorders had become the most costly diseases in the world. By then, another attempt at large-scale, cross-national epidemiologic surveys with improved diagnostic instruments had been initiated.[27]

Eventually, critics of the WHO's epidemiology proposed a combination of etic and emic methods to account for culture-bound standards of classification. The etic approach, according to the linguistic anthropologist Kenneth Pike, relies on extrinsic concepts and categories that have meaning for the scientific observer.[28] The methodology originally employed by the mental health experts at the WHO headquarters is a classic example of this philosophy, as it sought absolute objectivity and numerical rationality facilitated by advanced technology. In contrast, the emic perspective focuses on the intrinsic cultural distinctions that are meaningful to the members of a certain society. This approach has attracted psychiatric epidemiologists seeking to consider individuals' subjective perceptions. Since the 1960s, the epidemiologists of the Cornell School have been testing this combined approach.[29] Their work was once unpopular; however, these measures carry almost the same weight for psychiatric epidemiologists.

Psychiatry in the Two Chinas

Critiques of world standards for psychiatric diagnoses and disease profiles also emerged in Taiwan, the country that positioned itself as one of the best model students in the WHO's early decades. Tsung-yi Lin's student, Hsien Rin, argued that the confusion inherent in both the *ICD* and the *DSM* hindered psychiatric education and services. During a celebration of the twentieth anniversary of the Chinese Society of Neurology and Psychiatry, the psychiatric professional body based in Taiwan, he proposed a thorough discussion of the applicability of international standards, suggesting that the region should consider developing its own classification system.[30] Another Taiwanese psychiatrist, Keh-Ming Lin (1946–), who then taught at UCLA in the United States, expressed concern about Taiwan's role in producing academic knowledge. In an editorial in Taiwan's local psychiatry journal, he criticized scholars in Taiwan for validating the adaptability of theories and methods in developed countries while ignoring local needs. Clinical researchers in Taiwan, he argued, were unconcerned about local data. He asserted that scholars in Taiwan and other non-Western countries needed to develop their own visions and remain vigilant about their own cultures, to avoid establishing academic "export-processing zones" that were harmful to local populations.[31]

What was psychiatry like in the vast territory of China neglected by the WHO? Despite foundations laid by missionaries and tertiary education during the Republican period in China, modern psychiatry remained either a charitable or an academic enterprise in the post-World War II period.[32] In the 1950s, psychiatric services steadily grew in more than twenty provinces across the new People's Republic of China. Several epidemiological surveys were also conducted, covering a sample size of two to ten million in different studies, to provide a foundation for mental health planning.[33] These studies began well but stopped being conducted during the Cultural Revolution (1966–1976). During this period, mental health issues were neglected in the country, and psychiatric research was isolated. China was thus reluctant to help the field expand globally. During the initial phase of "reform and opening up," in the early 1980s, China experienced external pressure to adopt Western psychiatric theories and methods. Tsung-yi Lin, who had already left the WHO, was invited to advise China in developing its mental health project.[34] He published with Harvard psychiatrist Leon Eisenberg (1922–2009) a blueprint of mental health work for China, which tallied the state's planned economic proposals. Their book, *Mental Health Planning for One Billion People,* detailed existing mental health services and available epidemiological surveys on mental disorders in the early 1980s.[35] They also described the social factors in China that might have caused Chinese citizens' mental disturbances. At the time they made their proposal, psychiatry was still regarded with suspicion by most Chinese medical professionals. Notwithstanding their vision, no active plans were developed accordingly, partially because of Lin's later political agenda as an activist for Taiwan's independence despite his willingness to collaborate with the PRC, and partially because China needed a psychiatric system originating from within to account for its unique social, cultural, and political context.

That said, after having been separated from the rest of the world for so long, psychiatrists in China began to realize that they needed a valid classification system to account for the Chinese people's mental suffering. The *Chinese Classification of Mental Disorders* (*CCMD*), initially proposed to account for diseases observed only in a Chinese context, has undergone three major revisions since its first appearance in 1979.[36] In the early 1980s, the WHO agreed to help Chinese psychiatrists integrate the *CCMD* into the global system of classification,[37] and a collaborative research center for disease classification was established at Peking Union Medical Centre in 1981.[38] Yet, over four decades, gray areas have remained in the interpretation of mental symptoms, both cross-culturally and within China's state discourse.[39] Additional disease categories in the *CCMD* have accounted for sociocultural contexts, but unlike the ideologically based psychiatric taxonomy developed in Soviet Russia, the Chinese classifications have reflected an urgent need for new scientific instruments. For example, in the *CCMD-2,* "travel psychoses" appeared to be attributable to the worsening travel conditions on railways. It reflected the psychological backlash suffered by the Chinese during a period of accelerated economic growth, despite improved transportation infrastructure.[40] In 1994, the *CCMD-2R* definition of "induced psychosis," also known as *qigong piancha*, was created to account for psychological "deviations" associated with the practice of *qigong*, a system of physical exercises practiced in China that uses breathing control.[41] Such diagnoses, however, have been restricted to political purposes, such as being used to justify admitting Falun Gong practitioners to psychiatric hospitals, as human rights organizations reported in the 1990s.[42]

For the last three decades, the Chinese government and psychiatrists have been aware of the need to catch up with the world's standards regarding not only the quality of psychiatric services but the merit of academic research. Scholars have been carrying out epidemiological research to define the scope of China's psychiatric services and to develop mental health policies.[43] Following the method developed by the WHO, studies conducted in 1982 and 1983 used both *ICD* and *CCMD-2* classifications for disease. These studies concluded that the time point and lifetime prevalence of all mental disorders are 11.18% and 13.47%, respectively,[44] and that, apart from depression, the prevalence of major psychiatric disorders in China is similar to the WHO's findings. Depressive disorders, these studies found, are much less prevalent, yet as Arthur Kleinman observed, neurasthenia and depression have identical diagnoses in China, but neurasthenia manifests considerable somatic symptoms.[45] Not until the early twenty-first century, under the global power of the *DSM* system, did Chinese psychiatrists gradually replace the term "neurasthenia" with "subsyndromal depression" to respond to the practical needs in clinical practice and professional training that focused on making correct diagnoses.[46]

To improve its commitment to a public mental health infrastructure, China launched a series of projects in the 2000s that grew rapidly to cover the immense needs of more than one billion people. For example, the "686 Project" was launched in 2003, immediately after the devastation caused by the severe acute respiratory syndrome (SARS) epidemic. The project's goals were to reinforce community services, improve professional training, and construct a database of experiences to achieve successful reform.[47] In 2012, the nationwide China Mental Health Survey was implemented to analyze the overall state of mental health care. Leaders of the project had employed updated epidemiological survey tools commonly used by contemporary researchers in psychiatric epidemiology, including diagnostic instruments, such as the Composite International Diagnostic Interview and the Structured Clinical Interview, and diagnostic criteria for *DSM-IV*.[48]

Chinese pursuit of world standards was also reflected in its postsocialist public health governance. Figures obtained in the early 2000s became the parameters used in most research, with official documents estimating the numbers in need of psychiatric care as 17.5 million mentally ill individuals, 8.5 million of whom were diagnosed with schizophrenia.[49] Yet, as scholars of public health history have observed, state-sanctioned analyses imposed a positivist ideal, sought in the interests of social unity.[50] For example, in 2013, the health administration of Zhengzhou, a provincial capital in east-central China, asked local health offices to identify a mandatory 2 percent rate for severe psychiatric disorders, thereby increasing the risk of misdiagnoses and the potential for unjustifiable psychiatric admission.[51] From the 1980s onward, China's psychiatric research program has become subject to scrutiny at the WHO and elsewhere, but as this example shows, individuals may still fall victim to instrumental rationales in a system promoting metrical approaches.

Original Equipment Manufacturing for World Standards

How can we describe the relationship between the WHO and developing countries, or at least those who participated in its activities? International public health during the interwar period had consisted of a series of "administrative pilgrimages" shaped by preexisting ties such as the British imperial links among India, Burma, and Ceylon.[52] After World War II, public health programs replaced pilgrimages, and the WHO established a network of multiple interacting actors that followed a specific course. Accordingly, the Mental Health Unit's International Social Psychiatry Project was not merely an ideal put into practice but a complex system shaped by historical contingency. The WHO was a Cold War institutional bureaucracy, but it was also a transnational social network through which states and nonstate agents, including scientists, technocrats, and even technological artifacts, related to one another.

Historians have long argued about the structure of the WHO and the political factors that influenced its many projects. Most notable is Javed

Siddiqi's criticism of the organization's vertical model, which constrained the Malaria Eradication Program.[53] Commenting on Brock Chisholm's tenure at the WHO, John Farley cites early political disputes, after which Chisholm, who coined the phrase "world health" to replace "international health," left Geneva in July 1953. Frustrated that his desire for peace had been undermined, Chisholm lamented a world splitting into two powerful camps, one marked by the evils of Stalinism, the other by the madness of McCarthyism.[54] As Randall Packard recently argued, the WHO's hegemony in the international arena could expand its exercise of governmental power to large populations and, in some cases, secure "hearts and minds" against communism while making more people productive workers.[55]

As a transnational organization, the WHO also elicited uncertainties in some countries regarding their citizens' loyalty. For governments preferring that their citizens value membership in a nation state over world citizenship, the homogeneity of participating scientists was a major concern. For example, as Farley chronicles, in the early years of the WHO, the US wanted to screen its citizens employed by the WHO and other UN agencies for loyalty and asked them to sign loyalty oaths. Some of the WHO's participants did become openly critical of their governments' policies or opposed their governments' expressed interests.[56] Taiwan, for example, blacklisted Tsung-yi Lin for political reasons after he became a resistance leader against the Chinese Nationalist government during the early phases of the social psychiatry project. In 1972, working in the United States with two other scholars, he initiated the Self-Determination Movement for Taiwanese People. Lin henceforth experienced difficulties acquiring a visa and traveled internationally with a UN *laisser-passer* rather than a Taiwanese passport.[57] In addition to his pursuit of a career, Lin's moving to Geneva and then to North America gave him the freedom he had long desired. Such freedom was not only the freedom to travel but also the freedom from being constantly monitored by his home government.[58]

Political infighting and Cold War divisions could thus weaken programs in world health,[59] but scientists and doctors involved in mental health shared a belief in international collaboration and a vision of common metrics and a common language for research. Drawing from the genealogy of modern psychiatry, with its neo-Kraepelinian and neo-Freudian strands, the WHO recruited scientists committed to preventive medicine and new social measures, regardless of their school of psychiatry or their country of origin.

These scientists forged bonds with each other, even if they faced opposition at home, and maintained an esprit de corps that some scholars of science and technology characterize as a dreamscape (see chapter 5). Professionalism, in response to the devastation of World War II, further facilitated work on the WHO's projects and fed the tenacity of those who together shaped the social psychiatry project.

Unfortunately, despite the ideals of cross-national collaboration, the WHO's focus in the early postwar period remained Eurocentric. Despite efforts to include experts from non-Western regions or to conduct project seminars in non-Western countries, the vertical implementation of organizational policy meant that most developing countries simply tried to comply with standards set at headquarters. The result was an illusion of international harmony. The profile of schizophrenia, for example, became axiomatic across all participating countries. Mental disorders were reclassified and deemed universal. Discussion of culture-bound syndromes was suspended, even as these conditions were identified worldwide.

The WHO's headquarters operated like a company. Participating member states were like export-processing zones providing labor-intensive contributions to implement the WHO's projects from the periphery. This system of outsourcing has promoted cross-border production networks in industry since the 1960s; for example, IBM sought suppliers to manufacture personal computers with the company's technical assistance and its own technical design.[60] During the immediate post-World War II period, based on the notion that health could serve as a "magic bullet" to stimulate the growth of economies worldwide, especially in developing and underdeveloped countries, the WHO hoped to develop easy instruments to survey health and disease conditions and simple protocols for public health intervention.

Western and more developed countries, however, often underestimated public health achievements in developing countries, where medicalization and new infrastructures also facilitated the attainment of objectives.[61] For example, the WHO's grandest and the most extravagant effort was the Malaria Eradication Program. In many countries, successful eradication of malaria was not entirely the result of vertically imposed instructions from the WHO.[62] In Taiwan, eradication of malaria had begun earlier, but DDT spraying was extended for another two years, after its planned completion in 1956, to synchronize with the launch of the WHO's Malaria Eradication Program. Taiwan thus adapted its public health policies to meet the WHO's timeframes, to show its determination to work in concert with Geneva's project.[63]

If we look carefully at the so-called dreamscape of experts in developing countries, we also see an overemphasis on the importance of these experts' pursuit of world standards or an unwillingness to adjust to the ever-changing landscape in global health. Toward the end of the twentieth century, for example, Taiwan used its achievement in malaria eradication in its bid to rejoin the WHO, even though the organization had redirected its efforts to the control of infectious disease. Unsuccessful global eradication of malaria and polio are the classic cases. Mental health was no exception. In 1958, when the "manageable project" was still in development, China was the first of five priority countries believed to be in desperate need of development, but Lin thought Taiwan could make a significant contribution and so altered the WHO's priorities. Over the course of the International Social Psychiatry Project, new nation states, such as Israel, also sought to participate. The WHO thus adjusted its campaigns in response to flaws, drawbacks, and new developments.

A Culture-Bound *ICD*

Interestingly, as the WHO's Social Psychiatry Project was taking shape, researchers gradually identified a range of disorders consisting of unpredictable and chaotic behaviors, observable only in certain cultural settings. These disorders were first described by former Hong Kong-based psychiatrist Pow-Meng Yap as "atypical cultural bound psychogenic psychosis" but later abbreviated to "culture-bound syndromes."[64] Most of them had their roots in their historical contexts. But in the 1950s, the proliferating descriptions in psychiatric reports paved the way to the current view in the field of transcultural psychiatry. For example, the *Dhat* syndrome in India was characterized by vague psychosomatic symptoms and sexual dysfunction.[65] *Hwabyung*, another somaticized psychological distress expressed in a set of physical and anxiety-based complaints, was consistently described in South Korea and among overseas Korean communities.[66] Ancient *koro*, or penis-shrinking anxiety, related to the concerns of reproduction capacity among the Chinese, reappeared in Singapore and later outside Southeast Asia.[67] Latah, described by psychiatrists as a hyper-startle reaction, resulted in occurrences of imitation, cries, or violent behaviors in Malay and Javanese cultures.[68]

In Taiwan, on the other hand, disorders that initially attracted attention were marginalized, as Taiwan's psychiatry was linked to mainstream Anglo-American science. Taiwanese psychiatrists operating outside the scientific norm, however, promoted transcultural psychiatry. Lin's student Hsien Rin reported with him on conditions such as *hsieh-ping* and frigophobia among the Chinese, and *utox* among Taiwanese aboriginals. *Hsieh-ping* refers to a brief state during which one is possessed by an ancestral ghost; frigophobia is an unrealistic fear of becoming too cold that results in the person wearing heavy clothing. *Utox* is the processed state affected by the Atayal tribe's ancestral spirits. Another of Lin's students, Wen-Shing Tseng (1935–2012), lectured in Hawai'i for more than four decades and was celebrated for his renowned *Handbook of Cultural Psychiatry*.[69] Rin and Tseng developed their own schools of psychiatry, focusing on the effects of cultural differences on mental illnesses.[70] But these studies did not thoroughly explore the theoretical bases of disease nor clarify whether intrinsic biological (i.e., physical and mental) characteristics or extrinsic determinants of race determined manifestations of mental illnesses across cultures.

On the one hand, these discoveries—mainly in Asia, Latin America, and Africa—evoked colonial attitudes, as sufferers were often considered uncivilized. On the other hand, they implied the need for a pluralist psychiatry system. Their emergence pointed to the need for psychiatric attention to culture-specific conditions in non-Western countries. In the mid-1960s, scholars began to investigate culture-bound syndromes by combining methods from anthropology and epidemiology.[71] Anthropologists began to call for a "new cross-cultural psychiatry," propagated first by Arthur Kleinman in 1977, to study mental disorders in a way that respected cultural difference.[72] The discipline's continued heavy investment in the study of culture-bound syndromes included the "transcultural psychiatry" discipline initiated in the 1950s by Eric Wittkower and Jacob Fried. They gained repute through active correspondence with clinicians worldwide.[73] As discussed in chapter 2, in the 1960s through the refashioning of Henry B. M. Murphy and Raymond Prince (1925–2012), staff from the departments of psychiatry, sociology, and anthropology jointly established the Section of Transcultural Psychiatry at McGill University. To date, it remains the training hub to which interested psychiatric professionals flock to study the subject.[74] For the past half century, new accounts have claimed that definitions of normality and pathology should be derived only from local concepts, which cannot be generalized worldwide. Nonetheless, as sociologists Allan Horwitz and Jerome Wakefield argue, a universal human nature implies cross-cultural definitions of disease categories, including mental illness, which evolution would have distinguished from "the normal."[75]

As chapter 2 explains, however, cultural beliefs were subsumed under socioenvironmental stressors in the WHO's social psychiatry project, and in the ninth revision of the *ICD*, published in 1975, these syndromes were not included. Using changing disease categories as evidence, anthropologists have often criticized the definitions of psychiatric normality and abnormality as cultural constructs. In his book *Sickness and Healing: An Anthropological Perspective*, epidemiologist and anthropologist Robert Hahn argues that all diseases in the *ICD* system are both biological and cultural. Therefore, sociocultural factors independently cause illness, and all illnesses in the classification system are theoretically culture-bound.[76] However, in Hahn's words, "the [*ICD*] is a product of international collaboration, but collaborators have thus far all been trained in Biomedicine; traditional non-Biomedical medicines have not been represented."[77] The WHO's first social psychiatry project and its subsequent products, including revisions of the *ICD*, were bound to the short-lived ascendency of scientific internationalism and the organizational culture it promoted. Ironically, the knowledge it produced reflected the hegemony of knowledge still linked to a colonial past and imposed by a centrally planned system that is today criticized as having been hijacked by the pharmaceutical industry.

In the 1980s, the proposal to include culture-bound syndromes in the *ICD* or *DSM* systems reflected the profound ideological problem of defining universal diagnostic criteria for mental disorders. In psychiatry today, we are still asking whether a culturally sensitive diagnostic instrument is possible.[78] Scientists are still searching for methods that facilitate the understanding of mental disorders across cultures by reaching out to populations, such as immigrants, that are difficult to recruit to epidemiological studies. In certain clinical situations, cultural brokers are required to translate the styles and content of suffering into comprehensible symptoms. For the WHO, apart from revising the diagnostic system to facilitate dialogue with updated scientific research, revisions are expected to communicate with a more diverse population in primary care settings. To this end, achieving an international gold standard is a challenge, as the ways scientists imagine, understand, and classify mental disorders change with global culture.

Mobile Experts across the Globe

The recruitment of experts is one of the most important elements in the WHO's mode of knowledge production. Like its predecessor, the health office of the League of Nations, the WHO sought to attract health professionals from colonies (or former colonies) and to work with them as equals to those from the West. Technocratic efforts had similarly mobilized scientists to work together for a common purpose, but in several projects, collaborating experts faced uncertainty. The study group that looked at the mental health effect of atomic energy was one example (see chapter 2). Politics at the WHO, however, promoted the development of portable expertise in knowledge making and its dissemination across the globe. Because of the special conditions after World War II, science largely prevailed over the political obstacles and methodological critiques. The social psychiatry project thus succeeded in establishing a paradigm of worldwide collaboration in medical research.

Leaders at the WHO hoped their organizational design would surmount Cold War barriers to international collaboration. Fissures appeared elsewhere in the organization, however, as quarrels in the social psychiatry project occurred not along Cold War axes but among core members of the project. Experts from underdeveloped and developing countries were, in contrast, a homogeneous group, largely complying with instructions from Geneva. Early on, for example, some researchers did not agree that diseases other than schizophrenia could be studied by methods used for the IPSS,[79] but participants from peripheral countries did not question the validity of theories underlying the social psychiatry project. For them, the WHO offered a precious opportunity for small countries to be involved in a prestigious, large-scale international project, despite the fact that the WHO still remained a political stage for the postwar great powers.[80]

Recruiting likeminded psychiatrists who shared similar political visions and scientific backgrounds, the WHO could deploy experts beyond the *realpolitik* in international relations.[81] Although the collaborative work was planned in Geneva, the knowledge it produced exerted influence across the two major political blocs. The privilege of working at the WHO induced experts from various countries to apply their knowledge worldwide.[82] It also established a gold standard for several countries with underdeveloped mental health systems. After these scientists returned to their respective countries, they continued to work as clinicians, scientists, or technical advisors in different political, social, and cultural environments under the framework of the WHO.

National politics nonetheless complicated the work of the WHO's participating scientists. Some grew disillusioned with their own home countries and gradually detached themselves from their roles as scientific or technocratic advisors, often continuing to work as internationalists without formal ties to their home institutions.[83] For example, Tsung-yi Lin recalled in his memoir that he had learned methodologies such as the cluster analysis of data used at the FRC in Bethesda, Maryland, well enough to conduct research that attracted attention from all over the world.[84] After leaving the WHO, Lin applied what he had learned and continued to contribute to world health from affiliations in North America.[85] At home in Taiwan, however, his scientific contribution to local social psychiatry knowledge was never seen as being as important as his political campaigns, a side career he took upon returning to Taiwan after three decades of life abroad.

By association, modern psychiatry in postwar authoritarian states appeared to become provincialized. In the USSR and China, disease categories were designed to manage political dissidents.[86] In Taiwan, which was deemed a protectorate of the democratic bloc, Taiwanese psychiatrists were increasingly invited to participate in international mental health conferences. Their participation served two purposes. First, it facilitated the exchange of ideas and experiences between scholars from Taiwan and other countries. Second, for the Taiwanese government, sending delegates to international conferences served as a convenient method of monitoring international communism.[87] Individuals who wanted to attend medical conferences abroad were required to obtain permission from the Ministry of Foreign Affairs (MOFA) and from relevant authorities at the Chinese Nationalist Party Central Committee. Upon returning home, delegates were required to submit a report summarizing the conference, their contribution to it, experience and knowledge gained, the presence or absence of delegates from "pseudo-China," and the use of the official name Republic of China. For fear of propagating pro-Taiwan independence, MOFA forbade the use of "Taiwan" among delegates until the late 1980s. These local practices incongruously contradicted the objective of the WHO's principle of "the highest attainable level of health for all people."

Still One World, Many Cultures?

Local-global interactions shaped psychiatric epidemiology at the WHO. Local participation, however, was subject to the scrutiny of dominant Western countries,[88] so that the process was largely Eurocentric. As chapter 5 explains, the WHO and its member states engaged in a model of scientific collaboration. The model was originally established with "one world, many cultures" as its ideal framework but was better characterized as one heavy rope woven with too many strands.[89] Yet the relationship between headquarters and developing countries also approximated that of an international corporation and its export-processing zones. In these zones, subordinate laboratories contract with a dominant producer to manufacture products that meets its specifications. As the metaphor suggests, the input of experts from member states was not merely offering non-Western contributions to the social psychiatry project; rather, the WHO produced a reputable brand of postwar internationalism and attracted likeminded psychiatrists to carry out the visionary work of a few pioneers. Experts gathered in Geneva for numerous purposes, but a dreamscape motivated those from developing countries to join the enterprise. Their product was valuable but not as globally useful as many had expected.

The successes and limitations of the WHO's Social Psychiatry Project reflect broader changes at the organization. In 1960, the Mental Health Advisory panel comprised 70 psychiatric experts from 35 countries. During a speech at the International Congress on Mental Health in August 1961, Maria Pfister, the medical officer of the Mental Health Unit, noted an increase in UN member nations as new countries achieved independence, especially in Africa, and she reminded the audience that the WHO's work was complicated by the dynamics within the rapidly growing institution.[90] In the second half of the twentieth century, the Mental Health Unit, later restructured as the Mental Health Section or Department, became increasingly homogeneous as social scientists and anthropologists gradually withdrew and psychiatrists became the dominant professional community in global mental health.

The mental health work at the WHO also coincided with the formation of a new organization, the World Psychiatric Association (WPA), which emphasized nongovernmental leadership. In the 1960s, its members hotly debated abuses of psychiatry in certain countries, especially the USSR. The WHO, however, took no position on this issue, and the UN Secretariat had no response to the WPA's allegations of psychiatric abuse for political ends.[91] As with the development of nuclear weapons, the UN had little leverage for intervention. As the notable Japanese intellectual historian Shunsuke Tsurumi commented on postwar antinuclear attitudes, "As long as the world is conceived solely in terms of states, and people only as members of states, there can be little basis for criticizing the use of atomic bombs."[92] The same might be said of psychiatric practice.

The structure of the WHO was ideal for producing universally useful scientific knowledge. Postwar international relations played a major role in marshalling a staff of mobile experts who exemplified internationalist ideals through scientific collaboration. Initially, with the ethos of "the world helping the world," the highly political project intended both to produce greater prosperity and equity in the world and to prove that only international cooperation could produce the best results. In the social psychiatry project, therefore, downplaying cultural difference could ensure comparability among field research centers. Ignoring the Cold War could enhance the practicality of comparisons. In the end, even if the experts made international collaboration feasible, their accomplishment remained valid only in their mutually envisioned world.

Epilogue: Return to the Matrix

> If you can get on with people, bring people together, ... you can get things done, even when resources are minimal.
>
> Norman Sartorius (2019)

The second half of the twentieth century witnessed the globalization of mental health disorders. In the beginning, global health was a collective response to the desolation of war. Only gradually did psychiatrists become concerned with mental disorders that resulted from the effects of rapid socioeconomic development and the shifting boundaries between individuals and societies. Today, critiques of psychiatry focus on global medicalization and marketing by big pharmaceutical companies and other neoliberal engines. The biological foundation and symptom-based description of mental disorders are criticized for being the monotonous explanation of mental illness and for reducing human suffering into individualized pathology.[1] Yet, despite the century-long effort to trace the biological causes of mental disorders, a consensus still eludes scientists.[2] What is worse, alongside this pursuit is the globalization of psychiatric culture, which has influenced everyday life through the diffusion of commodities and ideas that promote standardization of cultural expression around the world.

This book has examined the prehistory of what we today term "global mental health," a concept that did not appear until the millennium. Global mental health is an initiative that seeks to detach itself from the hegemonic powers of "globalized psychiatry."[3] Many scholars got the definition wrong. If we look, however, at the quotation from the global mental health manifesto, "there can be no health without mental health,"[4] we might feel as though we are experiencing déjà vu because once again we come across the early WHO definition of health: "a state of complete physical, mental and social well-being and not merely the absence of disease or infirmity." Why should scientists reemphasize the significance of mental health? Are we repeating the same call? From the story told in this book, we can observe the subtle differences between the *Weltanschauungen* of postwar scientists who came from different belief systems and training backgrounds. In the immediate postwar period, scientists had placed their faith in an all-encompassing measure to understand mental disorders worldwide. But, unlike the criticism that the globalization of mental disorders was based on scientists' firm belief in biological psychiatry, the story presented in this book tells us that such a globalization process is interwoven with much more complex storylines that enabled a new practice of scientific knowledge production. These visionary scientists originally were calling for a bottom-up approach to mental disorders. They nevertheless failed to consider the accountability of such an approach in this complex and ever-changing world.

Having said that, however, I am not criticizing the WHO's International Social Psychiatry Project. In fact, the project has established a watershed in mental health research as a major program involving interlocking projects, research centers, and collaboration on a justly global level.[5] Besides, it stimulated debates and deliberation about an epistemologically relevant agenda. It has also invited us to rethink what we have taken for granted as "international," "world," and "global"—and what those terms have meant across different periods of contemporary history.

The movement of global mental health started in the 1990s with a group of psychiatrists looking cross-culturally at the need to scale up the accessibility of mental health services in the world. This problem was not foreseen by early WHO experts. Many critiques of this movement misunderstood its definition, assuming that due to its "global" label, the project was another hegemonic model of a mental health program. Therefore, the Edinburgh anthropologist Stefan Ecks emphasizes the importance of historicizing the resource, treatment, and credibility gaps between global mental health and local mental health.[6] David Satcher, the physician who coined the term, proposed that global mental health emphasized "partnership, mutual respect, and a shared vision of improving the lives of people who have mental illness and improving the mental health system for everyone."[7] Vikram Patel, the notable advocate of the global mental health initiative, emphasized a multidisciplinary approach to global mental health that harnesses the contributions of diverse fields of expertise, and advocated self-reflection in its practice.[8] The WHO's mental health projects, inaugurated soon after World War II, predated these appeals. In contrast with today's emphasis on local cultures, the WHO's early experts assumed there was universality in mental disorders. Applying a metrical approach, they worked across disciplines. The story of their efforts offers insights about contemporary problems in global mental health.

The previous incarnation of the concept of global mental health was the scientific knowledge and practice of international social psychiatry. Its construction was contingent on a universalist ideology, the operation of an overly ambitious international health organization, and optimism in technology. Most important, these high hopes were based on a scientific worldview shaped by cognitive, moral, and pragmatic ends in the second half of the twentieth century. The large-scale international effort at the WHO began long before the rise of global medical markets for pharmaceuticals when, in the immediate postwar period, scientists began to see mental disorders as universal. Rejecting colonial notions of racial inferiority, they envisioned universal criteria for diagnosing disease. No single individual tried to "invent" definitions of internationally valid mental disorders. Rather, a group of visionary scientists, influenced by the postwar ideological, political, and material environment, "imagined" mental disorders as global phenomena and, based on this vision, attempted to create metrics and identify manifestations and types of mental health conditions. The result was published in 1978 as chapter V of *ICD-9*. It was the culmination of decades of scientific collaboration but far from definitive. Instead, the quest to understand mental disorders continued, amid further deliberation.

Origins of the Gaps

Contemporary critiques aside, the zeal at the WHO to "globalize" mental disorders had little to do with the interests of pharmaceutical companies. In the mid-twentieth century, the WHO's scientists were focused on overcoming the devastation that afflicted populations had suffered in World War II. Theirs was a humanitarian intervention, not a desire to control. Like the spreading of *civitas* in the Roman Empire, a global system of mental health was to be an act of benevolent governance, without conquest, aimed at improvement in the lives of the governed.[9] For the WHO, the first objective was to understand mental disorders, conceived as public health problems, much like still-rampant infectious diseases. With utopian-like aspirations, a group of visionary psychiatrists thus set out to design a system that can be applied internationally on mental health care. Under the umbrella of the United Nations, they sought to prevent adversities in international public health.

But the contemporary gaps in global mental health had their origins. Planning a world-encompassing system was difficult in the Cold War era. The age of extremes extended to the assumed peacetime in which state nationalism and global capitalism grew. A number of areas remained colonized. Nonetheless, scientists based their collaboration on the notion of world citizenship and devised an innovative but complex structure to promote international collaboration. Its huge bureaucracy incorporated a system of outsourcing to experts who could work in accord with centrally defined methods. This design, I argue, was rooted in a specific international atmosphere and scientific vision. As an institution for the governance of global health, the WHO constituted a social world in which experts shared an idealistic yet quixotic worldview. To avoid a top-down approach, leaders of this collaborative project decentralized their research and recruited as many non-Western experts as possible. To produce universally usable knowledge, medical officers traveled and scientists participated in seminars worldwide.

For the WHO, scientific knowledge relied on several historical contingencies. First, by regarding mental disorders as diseases amenable to intervention in public health, psychiatrists took nearly two decades to establish their discipline as mainstream medicine supported by quantitative validation. Second, methodology that regarded culture as a social determinant instead of an intrinsic quality of mind enabled scientists to compare their data. Scientific internationalists and cultural relativists thus met on common ground, where they could together refute colonial-era ideas of race and hierarchy. Third, the zeal to create metrics under the idea of standardization promoted a technological turn, supported by the development of videotaping and computing. The profiling and classification of mental disorders was both advanced and limited by these technologies.

Global-local interactions shaped psychiatric epidemiology at the WHO, with survey studies at the international level. The relationship between Geneva and participating countries represented neither the dominance of the Global South by the Global North nor a trading zone in which participants from different backgrounds exchanged views and plans. Rather, experts shared a dreamscape of decentralized collaboration. A shared vision and common scientific background linked planners in the Geneva headquarters with experts from developing member states. In Taiwan, for example, mental health surveys were developed to promote national autonomy and provided a deracialized design for conducting research. With the surveys, Taiwanese scientists sought involvement in global health and further forged international bonds. Their aspiration, however, was a momentary dream that universally defined mental disorders could be measurable, comparable, and perhaps treatable worldwide.

"Outsourcing," rather than "globalizing," more accurately describes the WHO's structural design. Outsourcing was a strategy to prevent the implementation of a top-down protocol, but homogeneity among experts made the social psychiatry project resemble the system of original equipment manufacturing, common in some industries, in which a brand-name company outsources its specifications to smaller, lesser-known producers. Although experts recruited to the system showed their passion about the WHO's work, it is hard to say that they represented their own culture. Instead, their similar training made them convenient individuals for collaboration with Geneva's core team. In this model, developing countries participated not by contributing local knowledge to headquarters, but by following the instruction manual written at the headquarters without bestowing much of their own expertise. The research paradigm of the IPSS and *ICD-9* laid important foundations for international psychiatric epidemiology, but their designs were ultimately criticized for flawed representation and other sampling errors in some populations.

The Undetermined Future of Mental Health Standards

Is the WHO's model of international collaboration no longer worth promoting? Do we need a common language for international mental health? This book addresses these questions by telling a story largely unknown among psychiatric practitioners, advocates, and researchers today. At one historical moment, a group of experts joined an institution and developed a project on a global scale to model international collaboration and to identify the errors and obstacles a large-scale project might encounter. Today, their efforts show that the function of scientific knowledge can vary over time and space. After the 1970s, for example, the relationship between the WHO and its member states changed significantly, and Geneva began to respond strategically to member state demands.[10] This shift stemmed in part from economic development and a growing middle class in developing countries.[11] The work the experts did clearly solved a wide range of disease problems in these countries. This narrative points as well to the difficulties of producing all-encompassing health policies in a world that has become more complex.

In the 1970s, the WHO's approach to mental health saw a turn from internationalism and planning to need-based strategies. Observers and practitioners in Southeast Asia identified the immense difficulty of creating and implementing effective psychiatric therapeutic systems. Before clinical psychiatry could be developed, the failure to provide basic services to the populations of developing countries was the major obstacle to overcome.[12] Difficulties also existed on other levels: the socioeconomic capability of developing countries to attain the essential standards of modern care, community acceptability of psychiatric facilities, and efforts to accommodate cultural needs and customs.[13] In 1978, with participation from virtually all member states of the WHO and UNICEF, the International Conference on Primary Health Care convened in Alma-Ata, Kazakhstan. The Alma-Ata Declaration signed during the conference became a milestone in public health that emphasized primary health care as the foundation of the goal, defined by the WHO, of "the highest attainable level of health for all people." Mental health experts' awareness of such a need had emerged earlier. In 1975, represented by Norman Sartorius, T. W. Harding, and Joy Moser, the WHO's Mental Health Office had outlined priorities for wide-scale service intervention, including psychiatric auxiliaries, group therapy, village settlements, and rural outpatient clinics.[14] The report published by the Mental Health Expert Committee in 1975 recommended that member states in developing countries decentralize health services, integrate mental health care with general health practices, and allow mental health tasks to be shared among psychiatrists and a wider range of health workers and community agencies.[15] While a new era of mental health policy thus unfolded, African and Latin American countries entered upon the stage. In the case of Taiwan and China, as discussed in chapters 4 and 6, their zealous pursuit of international standards and universal metrical approaches, in either clinical services or scientific research, seems to have prevented them from participating in the most recent global mental health movement, which focuses on more basic and substantive needs among mentally disturbed people.

From the emergence of humanitarian intervention to the shaping of global mental health, experts at the WHO did not anticipate the consequences of their work. While their project was taking shape, they failed to foresee that interdisciplinary collaboration would gradually be subjugated by the single profession of modern psychiatry. They did not realize that the science they pursued would support some ideologies but neglect others. Entering the twenty-first century, global mental health keeps evolving, with multiple genealogies. Apart from its qualitative turn away from conventional international health and development, it has become the project of various professional networks and social movements. Nevertheless, it has also been criticized for becoming a diagnostically oriented and metrics-driven psychiatric imperialism enabled by big pharma.[16] As noted by medical anthropologist Didier Fassin, while "worldwide" is geographical and proposes a mere description of observed facts, "universal" is ideological and suggests a form of claimed hegemony, implying superiority.[17] By creating universal metrics, these experts pursued neutrality, but their international language and organizational infrastructure acquired characteristics of empire and promoted the global reach of pharmaceutical companies. In their quest for a universal standard, they imagined a world connected through science, which could offer the imprimatur of inclusion.

Imagination in science is a response to social and cultural contexts. Much as C. Wright Mills elaborates a "sociological imagination," scientists link their own experience to the wider society. This scientific imagination not only offers a perspective for understanding the world but also informs scientists' commitments in knowledge production. Between the immediate post-World War II period and the early twenty-first century, the way scientists imagined the world changed. So did the way psychiatrists imagined mental disorders and the discipline of psychiatry. The desire for a standard and method for apprehending mental disorders receded. In a world marked by greater ideological heterogeneity and a widening gap between rich and poor, mental health experts are focusing on better provision of services. As Erich Fromm asserted, "mental health cannot be defined in terms of the 'adjustment' of the individual to his society, but, on the contrary, ... it must be defined in terms of the adjustment of the society to the needs of man."[18] The trajectory of global mental health suggests a future that will unquestionably be different.

In its first decades, the WHO moved from its position as the unquestioned leader of international health to an organization in crisis, facing budget shortfalls and weakened status.[19] Its problems were caused not only by the growing influence of new and powerful players in health governance but also by a change in the ways that diseases and health are comprehended. Unlike the past concern about the absence of mental health resources in underdeveloped countries, today's focus stems from observations that individuals with mental disorders, such as schizophrenia, who live in less developed countries enjoy better outcomes than their Western counterparts. This finding corroborates results of the WHO's 1992 DOSMED study, which confused researchers. In some developing countries, patients and family members are either undiagnosed or underdiagnosed, and individuals may be labeled with disorders that permeate their everyday life.[20] This situation provokes a question: Might global health be better without a globally standardized diagnostic system? With the revision of the new *ICD* system, together with the global trend of promoting primary care, came calls to emphasize the system's clinical utility rather than the validity of standardized metrics.[21]

In addition, as the WHO began to reshape its strategy, its leaders recognized the need for alternative methods of knowledge production and a more democratic system of governance. In response to a globalizing economy, some voices have advocated an "alter-globalization" that focuses on global cooperation and interaction among nongovernment organizations and activists instead of the conventional knowledge transfer such as dissemination or diffusion.[22] As the *ICD* was revised, for example, the task force considered the suggestions of users, in contrast to the elite approach of the US-based *DSM* system. A recent debate about whether to remove the chapter on gender incongruence disorder in childhood provided one dilemma.[23] Mental health professionals lamented the conundrum they faced between the stigma of a diagnosis and the lack of treatment for patients who lacked a diagnosis. Based on users' experiences, calls have thus been made to redefine best practices by responding to the grounded needs and human rights of vulnerable populations.[24] In the most recently published *ICD-11*, the long-debated gender incongruence disorder was moved out of the chapter on mental disorders and into the chapter on sexual health conditions.[25]

Moreover, a gaming disorder entered the global scene after China first ratified the need to diagnose suffering teenagers.[26] As this book shows, such conundrums occur not only for specific diagnoses but also in the ways diagnoses are transnationally imagined, manufactured, and negotiated among various stakeholders.

The past half century has seen a collective trend to create universal metrics for understanding mental disorders. As medical historian Robert Aronowitz put it, metrics are the object of idiosyncrasy among scientists.[27] And now we have arrived at a critical moment in which the WHO's member states are trying simultaneously to increase adoption of the *ICD* and to focus on the sociocultural matrix in which mental disorders are shaped, understood, and managed. The early thrust for standardized approaches to mental disorders placed competing demands for international comparability against national needs (e.g., representative official statistics).[28] We might therefore question whether space remains for rethinking the idea of universal mental disorders. A nuanced historical understanding can inform any such consideration. History can help explain the contributions of the WHO's organizational processes to its system and can inform psychiatrists worldwide who have been seeking refined and subtle understanding of mental disorders. Today, disciplines negotiate management of the global burden of mental health in a pluralist society, which the world has gradually become.

The findings of this book reflect a remark of Professor Norman Sartorius, who continued Tsung-yi Lin's work at the WHO. Commenting on epidemiology and the development of a common language, he stated, "In the past 20 years, the rapid appearance of new technologies had caused our delay in accumulating adequate data, in order to help us verify the evidence supporting the concepts and entities of diseases." He further noted that "The growing distance between neuroscientists, clinicians and epistemologists has also created problems."[29] As Assen Jablensky, the Australian psychiatric nosologist, who has been participating in the WHO's classification project, asserted, disease classification is a complex matter. It reflects both the achievements and the conflicts in the development of modern psychiatry.

ICD-11 was published in June 2018, three years after it was supposed to be on bookshelves, a delay perhaps due to the complexity of a more deliberative process of knowledge making. The revision reduced the number of disease categories to simplify treatment.[30] In 2012, *DSM-5*, published in the United States, instead located mental diseases across the wide spectrum of human psychology. Its complexity presented problems in clinical application, and critics decried the interests of pharmaceutical companies and other groups. Yet, as Kenneth Kendler, a member of the *DSM-5* task force, pointed out, the design of the new classification system was dimensional instead of categorical. This principle corresponds with the concept of "iteration" raised by philosopher of science Hasok Chang, who described an iterative system as a mathematical method that pursues not a single solution but several approximate solutions and can repeatedly self-correct to accommodate new information.[31] This new paradigm—without recourse to arbitrary scientific measurement—is expected to meet the demands of ever-changing modern society. These efforts are just a part of the agenda of such experts as the Mental Health Gap Action Program, the global mental health movement, and numerous psychosocial support schemes.

Hearing Echoes from the Past

In the mid-twentieth century, a way of thinking and a common language, based on a utopian ideology, were established by a brave institution with a new kind of science and promising technology. At that time, such thinking emerged as a binary between universality and cultural disparities. In fact, the story presented in this book tells us that negotiation between these perspectives had emerged when scientists started to cast doubt and look for methods to confirm whether such a binary really existed. In addition, it was the notion of human equality that guided the manufacturing of this common language, but gradually and unexpectedly such common language became a system of imperial governance, reaching into people's everyday lives. In the early postwar period, however, the idealistic notion of world citizenship infused international collaboration in scientific research. Science, its proponents claimed, could establish the basis for human equality.

Today, researchers in mental health have abandoned the a priori of the global community as a single ethnicity, and have instead discussed subjective experiences and the cultural construction of selves. This aspect of global mental health research has been corroborated by anthropological studies worldwide. As anthropologist Aihwa Ong argues, globalization has led not to the "denationalization of citizenship" but to "specific articulations between national citizenship and transnational norms." This cultural specificity also promoted the growth of nonstate spaces where transnational institutions could intervene on grounds of humanity rather than citizenship.[32] Now that the heterogeneous world has become so different from the united world that was imagined during the immediate postwar period, how will our ever-changing worldview alter social psychiatry and psychiatric classification? How are bureaucratic, slow-responding international organizations that serve the status quo going to transform their structures and *modi operandi*? Will artificial intelligence facilitate or obstruct scientific research? None of these questions can be answered by this book. Here, however, is a historical reference for mental health workers, either clinical or nonclinical, to develop more contextual awareness and culturally sensitive skills while facing mental suffering.

In science, we often believe that we are empiricists championing scientific methods through experimentation with shared objectives. With scientific findings resting on evidence, the pursuit of knowledge becomes an agenda for research. Retrospectively, however, research agendas are imagined, temporal constructs full of unexpected developments, full stops, and restarts. Unconscious biases can sometimes influence objectives or interpretations of evidence, and evidence deemed solid might also become invalid when values change. I recall my first archival trip to Geneva, where a young intern at the WHO shared with me her excitement at working with an important NGO, which she assumed was focused on doing good. At the time, I was similarly naïve, seeking to tell the story of Tsung-yi Lin, who is much celebrated in Taiwan but otherwise largely unknown. Now, I realize, Lin's transnational project transcended individuals and disciplines but was at the same time constrained by the postwar era. Responding to a legacy of war and colonial oppression, the experts he oversaw sought collaboratively to conceptualize and classify mental disorders. The desiderata have never been completed. We are still sailing with a world map of knowledge that has never been accurately drawn.

I hope that this book will be significant to historians and sociologists of science, technology, and medicine and thought-provoking for clinicians. I hope too that, drawing from different perspectives on health and diseases, this story can benefit public discussion and inform researchers and planners of global mental health. More important, I hope that the public recognizes the ways in which a context-bound imagination drives scientists forward, despite the world's discontents. Perhaps, then, we may perceive the limitations of a world that falls short of the utopia we were promised by science.

Archives

The Alan Mason Chesney Medical Archives of the Johns Hopkins Medical Institutions, Baltimore, Maryland, USA

The Bethlem Museum of the Mind, Beckenham, Kent, UK
Aubrey Lewis Personal Papers

The British Society of Psychoanalysis, London, UK
John Bowlby P25A, P25B

King's College London, London, UK
Aubrey Lewis Papers

The London School of Hygiene and Tropical Medicine, London, UK
Donald Reid Papers

The National Archives of the United Kingdom, Kew, London
Foreign Offices
National Association of Mental Health

The National Institutes of Health, Bethesda, Maryland, USA
Robert Felix Papers

Queen Mary, University of London, London, UK
Eileen Brooke Papers PP32

The Wellcome Library, London, UK
John Bowlby Papers

World Health Organization, Geneva, Switzerland
Director-General Offices
Mental Health: M4; WHO/MENT (Microfiche)

Notes

Chapter 1

1. Vincanne Adams, "Metrics of the Global Sovereign: Numbers and Stories in Global Health," in *Metrics: What Counts in Global Health*, ed. Vincanne Adams (Durham: Duke University Press, 2016), 19–54.

2. In this book, I use "mental disorders" as a general designation to refer to diseases of mental or behavioral patterns that cause individual suffering and malfunctioning. These conditions are also known as "mental illnesses" or "psychiatric disorders" in different contexts. In anthropological terms, illness, disease, and disorder might have different meanings. Here, however I apply the term "mental disorders" to avoid confusion. Other terms do, of course, appear in quotations and analysis of others' scholarship.

3. Andrew Scull, *Madness in Civilization* (Princeton, NJ: Princeton University Press, 2015). See also Allen Frances, *Saving Normal: An Insider's Revolt against Out-of-Control Psychiatric Diagnosis, DSM-5, Big Pharma, and the Medicalization of Ordinary Life* (New York: William Morrow, 2013).

4. Thomas Insel, "Transforming Diagnosis," *National Institute of Mental Health*, posted on April 29, 2013, https://www.nimh.nih.gov/about/directors/thomas-insel/blog/2013/transforming-diagnosis.shtml.

5. Frances, *Saving Normal*, 18–23, 79–81.

6. WHO Archive, M4/445/2(e).

7. World Health Organization, *Manual of the International Statistical Classification of Diseases, Injuries, and Causes of Death: Sixth Revision of the International Lists of Diseases and Causes of Death, Adopted 1948*, Bulletin of the World Health Organization: Supplement, 2 vols. (Geneva: World Health Organization, 1948).

8. Assen Jablensky, "Psychiatric Classifications: Validity and Utility," *World Psychiatry* 15, no. 1 (February 2016): 26–31, https://doi.org/10.1002/wps.20284.

9. L. J. Kirmayer, "Beyond the 'New Cross-Cultural Psychiatry': Cultural Biology, Discursive Psychology and the Ironies of Globalization," *Transcultural Psychiatry* 42, no. 1 (March 2006): 126–144.

10. Richard Horton, "Launching a New Movement for Mental Health," *The Lancet* 370, no. 9590 (September 4, 2007): 806.

11. Tsung-Mei Cheng, "Taiwan's National Health Insurance System: High Value for the Dollar," in *Six Countries, Six Reform Models: The Healthcare Reform Experience of Israel, The Netherlands, New Zealand, Singapore, Switzerland and Taiwan; Healthcare Reform "Under the Radar Screen,"* ed. Kieke G. H. Okma and Luca Crivelli (Singapore: World Scientific, 2009), 171–204.

12. Megan Greene, *The Origins of the Developmental State in Taiwan: Science Policy and the Quest for Modernization* (Cambridge, MA: Harvard University Press, 2008).

13. C. G. Seligman, "Temperament, Conflict and Psychosis in a Stone-Age Population," *Psychology and Psychotherapy* 9, no. 3 (1929): 187–202.

14. Sing Lee, "Cultures in Psychiatric Nosology: The CCMD-2-R and International Classification of Mental Disorders," *Culture, Medicine and Psychiatry* 20, no. 4 (1996): 421–472.

15. Sing Lee, "From Diversity to Unity: The Classification of Mental Disorders in 21st-Century China," *Psychiatric Clinics* 24, no. 3 (2001): 521–431.

16. *Hiroshima Mon Amour*, dir. Alain Resnais, screenplay by Marguerite Duras (Paris: Argos-Films, 1959), DVD. Also see Marguerite Duras, *Hiroshima Mon Amour*, trans. Richard Seaver (New York: Grove Press, 1961), 15–16.

17. Despo Kritsotaki, Vicky Long, and Matthew Smith, eds., *Deinstitutionalisation and After: Post-War Psychiatry in the Western World* (London: Palgrave Macmillan, 2016).

18. Executive Board, Expert Committee on Mental Health, Seventh Report (Social Psychiatry and Community Attitudes), World Health Organization, 24th session, May 23, 1959, http://www.who.int/iris/handle/10665/135276.

19. See Byron Good and Mary-Jo Delvecchio Good, "Significance of the 686 Program for China and for Global Mental Health," *Shanghai Archives of Psychiatry* 24, no. 3 (2012): 175–177; and Arthur Kleinman, *Rethinking Psychiatry: From Cultural Category to Personal Experience* (New York: Free Press, 1988).

20. Sigmund Freud, *Civilization and Its Discontents* (London: Hogarth Press, 1953), 141–142.

21. See Thomas Szasz, *Medicalization of Everyday Life: Selected Essays* (Syracuse, NY: Syracuse University Press, 2007).

22. Robert Whitaker, *Anatomy of an Epidemic: Magic Bullets, Psychiatric Drugs, and the Astonishing Rise of Mental Illness in America* (New York: Crown Publishers, 2010).

23. Gary Greenberg, *The Book of Woe: The DSM and the Unmaking of Psychiatry* (New York: Blue Rider Press, 2013).

24. Michael E. Staub, *Madness Is Civilization: When the Diagnosis Was Social, 1948–1980* (Chicago: University of Chicago Press, 2015); Ethan Watters, *Crazy Like Us: The Globalization of the American Psyche* (New York: Free Press, 2010).

25. Bruce M. Z. Cohen, *Psychiatric Hegemony: A Marxist Theory of Mental Illness* (London: Palgrave Macmillan, 2016).

26. China Mills, *Decolonizing Global Mental Health: The Psychiatrization of the Majority World* (New York: Routledge, 2014); China Mills, "Global Psychiatrization and Psychic Colonization: The Coloniality of Global Mental Health," in *Critical Inquiries for Social Justice in Mental Health*, ed. Marina Morrow and Lorraine Halinka Malcoe (Toronto: University of Toronto Press, 2017), 87–109.

27. Erich Fromm, *The Sane Society* (New York: Holt, Rinehart and Winston, 1955), 14–15.

28. Ibid., 12.

29. Richard Horton, "Offline: Frantz Fanon and the Origins of Global Health," *The Lancet* 392, no. 10149 (September 1, 2018): 720, https://doi.org/10.1016/S0140-6736(18)32041-5.

30. See Kritsotaki, Long, and Smith, *Deinstitutionalisation and After*; and Staub, *Madness Is Civilization*.

31. James Belich, John Darwin, Margret Frenz, and Chris Wickham, *The Prospect of Global History* (Oxford: Oxford University Press, 2016).

32. Mark Harrison, "A Global Perspective: Reframing the History of Health, Medicine, and Disease," *Bulletin of the History of Medicine* 89, no. 4 (2015): 639–689.

33. Mark Harrison, *Contagion: How Commerce Has Spread Disease* (New Haven: Yale University Press, 2012).

34. Akira Iriye, *Global Community: The Role of International Organizations in the Making of the Contemporary World* (Berkeley: University of California Press, 2002).

35. Glenda Sluga, *Internationalism in the Age of Nationalism* (Philadelphia: University of Pennsylvania Press, 2013).

36. Bruce Mazlish and Akira Iriye, *The Global History Reader* (New York: Routledge, 2005).

37. Sunil S. Amrith, "Internationalising Health in the Twentieth Century," in *Internationalisms: A Twentieth-Century History*, ed. Glenda Sluga (Cambridge: Cambridge University Press, 2017), 245–264.

38. *Article XXIII, Treaty of Peace with Germany, Hearings before the Committee on Foreign Relations, United States Senate, Sixty-sixth Congress, First Session* (Washington: Government Printing Office, 1919), 275.

39. Iriye, *Global Community*, vii.

40. Marcos Cueto, Theodore M. Brown, and Elizabeth Fee, "The Birth of the World Health Organization, 1945–1948," in *The World Health Organization: A History* (Cambridge: Cambridge University Press, 2019), 34–61.

41. Waltraud Ernst and Thomas Müller, *Transnational Psychiatries: Social and Cultural Histories of Psychiatry in Comparative Perspective, c. 1800–2000* (Newcastle: Cambridge Scholars, 2010), xi.

42. Ibid., iv.

43. Ibid., viii.

44. Volker Roelcke, Paul Weindling, and Louise Westwood, *International Relations in Psychiatry: Britain, Germany, and the United States to World War II* (Rochester, NY: University of Rochester Press, 2010).

45. For instance, "Historicizing Transcultural Psychiatry," special issue, *History of Psychiatry* 29, no. 3 (September 2018), https://journals.sagepub.com/toc/hpya/29/3.

46. "Psychology and Psychiatry in the Global World, Part I," special issue, *History of Psychology* 22, no. 3 (August 2019), https://www.apa.org/pubs/journals/special/5582205.

47. In John Farley, *Brock Chisholm, the World Health Organization, and the Cold War* (Vancouver: University of British Columbia Press, 2008), 90.

48. This common omission was pointed out by Hannah S. Decker, *The Making of DSM-III: A Diagnostic Manual's Conquest of American Psychiatry* (New York: Oxford University Press, 2013).

49. World Health Organization, *The First Ten Years of the World Health Organization* (Geneva: World Health Organization, 1958); World Health Organization, *The Second Ten Years of the World Health Organization* (Geneva: World Health Organization, 1968); Socrates Litsios and World Health Organization, *The Third Ten Years of the World Health Organization, 1968–1977* (Geneva: World Health Organization, 2008).

50. Mills, *Decolonizing Global Mental Health.*

51. For example, see Sunil S. Amrith, *Decolonizing International Health: India and Southeast Asia, 1930–65* (Basingstoke: Palgrave Macmillan, 2006). For a recent mental health agenda, see Mills, *Decolonizing Global Mental Health.*

52. Harold Maurice Collins, "The Sociology of Scientific Knowledge: Studies of Contemporary Science," *Annual Review of Sociology*, no. 9 (1983): 265–285.

53. Harry Collins and Robert Evans, *Rethinking Expertise* (Chicago: University of Chicago Press, 2007).

54. However, these projects are different from the "international social psychiatry movement" irregularly promoted by socialist psychiatrists in the 1960s, although

some propagators, such as Aubrey Lewis, overlapped with the WHO's work. See Liam Clarke, "Joshua Bierer: Striving for Power," *History of Psychiatry* 8, no. 31 (September 1997): 319–332; Mat Savelli, "Beyond Ideological Platitudes: Socialism and Psychiatry in Eastern Europe," *Palgrave Communication* 4, no. 45 (2018).

55. Farley, *Brock Chisholm.*

56. Peter Galison, *Image and Logic: A Material Culture of Microphysics* (Chicago: University of Chicago Press, 1997); Sheila Jasanoff and Sang-Hyun Kim, *Dreamscapes of Modernity: Sociotechnical Imaginaries and the Fabrication of Power* (Chicago: University of Chicago Press, 2015).

57. John Krige, ed., *How Knowledge Moves: Writing the Transnational History of Science and Technology* (Chicago: University of Chicago Press, 2019).

58. Assen Jablensky and Norman Sartorius, "What Did the WHO Study Really Find?," *Schizophrenia Bulletin* 34, no. 2 (2008): 253–255.

59. See Hasok Chang, *Inventing Temperature: Measurement and Scientific Progress* (Oxford: Oxford University Press, 2007), 44–48; also Kenneth S. Kendler, "Epistemic Iteration as a Historical Model for Psychiatric Nosology: Promises and Limitations," in Kenneth S. Kendler and Josef Parnas, eds., *Philosophical Issues in Psychiatry II: Nosology* (Oxford: Oxford University Press, 2012), 305–322.

Chapter 2

1. Marcos Cueto, Theodore M. Brown, and Elizabeth Fee, *The World Health Organization: A History* (Cambridge: Cambridge University Press, 2019), 44.

2. See Javed Siddiqi, *World Health and World Politics: The World Health Organization and the UN System* (Columbia: University of South Carolina Press, 1995).

3. John Farley, *Brock Chisholm, the World Health Organization, and the Cold War* (Vancouver: University of British Columbia Press, 2008).

4. Cueto, Brown, and Fee, *The World Health Organization*, 58.

5. Steve Sturdy, Richard Freeman, and Jennifer Smith-Merry, "Making Knowledge for International Policy: WHO Europe and Mental Health Policy, 1970–2008," *Social History of Medicine* 26, no. 3 (2013): 532–554.

6. Michael D. Gordin, *Scientific Babel: How Science Was Done Before and After Global English* (Chicago: University of Chicago Press, 2015).

7. Glenda Sluga, *Internationalism in the Age of Nationalism* (Philadelphia: University of Pennsylvania Press, 2013), 12–13.

8. Paul Forman, "Scientific Internationalism and the Weimar Physicists: The Ideology and Its Manipulation in Germany after World War I," *Isis* 64, no. 2 (June 1973):

150–180; Paul Weindling, "The 'Sonderweg' of German Eugenics: Nationalism and Scientific Internationalism," *British Journal for the History of Science* 22, no. 3 (September 1989): 321–333.

9. John Krige, "Atoms for Peace, Scientific Internationalism, and Scientific Intelligence," *Osiris* 21, no. 1 (2006): 161–181; Clark A. Miller, "An Effective Instrument of Peace: Scientific Cooperation as an Instrument of U.S. Foreign Policy, 1938–1950," *Osiris* 21, no. 1 (2006): 133–160; and Eric Bennett, *Workshops of Empire: Stegner, Engle, and American Creative Writing during the Cold War* (Iowa City: University of Iowa Press, 2015).

10. Akira Iriye, *Cultural Internationalism and World Order* (Baltimore: Johns Hopkins University Press, 2000).

11. Bennett, *Workshops of Empire*, 67.

12. "About the WHO," *World Health Organization* webpage.

13. Cueto, Brown, and Fee, *The World Health Organization*, 44.

14. Although the term "global" did not emerge to replace "international" and embrace a much wider scope of concerns until recently.

15. See Ben Shephard, *A War of Nerves: Soldiers and Psychiatrists, 1914–1994* (London: Pimlico, 2002); Edgar Jones and Simon Wessely, *Shell Shock to PTSD: Military Psychiatry from 1900 to the Gulf War* (Hove, UK: Psychology Press, 2005); Allan Young, *The Harmony of Illusions: Inventing Post-traumatic Stress Disorder* (Princeton, NJ: Princeton University Press, 1995).

16. Herbert Allen Carroll, *Mental Hygiene: The Dynamics of Adjustment* (Englewood Cliffs, NJ: Prentice-Hall, 1964).

17. Dagmar Herzog, *Cold War Freud: Psychoanalysis in an Age of Catastrophes* (New York: Cambridge University Press, 2017).

18. Mark Jackson, *The Age of Stress: Science and the Search for Stability* (New York: Oxford University Press, 2013), 141–180.

19. Naoko Wake, *Private Practices: Harry Stack Sullivan, the Science of Homosexuality, and American Liberalism* (New Brunswick, NJ: Rutgers University Press, 2011), 325–338.

20. Shephard, *A War of Nerves*, 163–168.

21. John R. Rees, *The Shaping of Psychiatry by War* (New York: Academy of Medicine; London: Chapman and Hall, 1945), 115.

22. Wake, *Private Practices*, 163–168.

23. Alan Gregg, "The Limitations of Psychiatry," *American Journal of Psychiatry* 104, no. 9 (1948): 513–522.

24. Kenneth Soddy to William Moodie, May 27, 1946, Wellcome Archives SA/BMA /B.87.

25. Farley, *Brock Chisholm.*

26. George Brock Chisholm, *Prescription for Survival* (New York: Columbia University Press, 1957), 92.

27. British Psychoanalytical Society Archive P25-A-01.

28. Jonathan Kahana and Noah Tsika, "*Let There Be Light* and the Military Talking Picture," in *Remaking Reality: U.S. Documentary Culture after 1945*, ed. Sara Blair, Joseph B. Entin, and Franny Nudelman (Chapel Hill: University of North Carolina Press, 2018), 14–34.

29. As William Menninger disclosed during the first postwar gathering of the American Psychiatric Association (APA) in 1946, close to two million men were rejected for military service during the war as a result of "neuropsychiatric disorders," and an additional one million had become "neuropsychiatric admissions" to army hospitals in the years from 1942 to 1945. Cited in Michael E. Staub, *Madness Is Civilization: When the Diagnosis Was Social, 1948–1980* (Chicago: University of Chicago Press, 2015), 20.

30. See Gerald N. Grob, *From Asylum to Community* (Princeton, NJ: Princeton University Press, 2014). Japanese psychiatrists also held dichotomized attitudes; see Ran Zwigenberg, *Hiroshima: The Origins of Global Memory Culture* (Cambridge: Cambridge University Press, 2014).

31. Karl M. Bowman, "Presidential Addresses," *American Journal of Psychiatry* 103, no. 1 (July 1946): viii, 1–17.

32. Donald Ewen Cameron, "Presidential Addresses: Psychiatry and Citizenship," *American Journal of Psychiatry* 110, no. 1 (1953): xii, 2–9. Cameron later became the founding president of the World Psychiatric Association in 1961. He is, however, nowadays more controversial because of his mysterious involvement in the CIA's MK-Ultra Project, which aimed to "brainwash" communists during the Korean War. See Rebecca Lemov, *World as Laboratory: Experiments with Mice, Mazes, and Men* (New York: Hill and Wang, 2005).

33. Sunil S. Amrith, *Decolonizing International Health: India and Southeast Asia, 1930–65* (Basingstoke: Palgrave Macmillan, 2006).

34. Daniel Pick, *The Pursuit of the Nazi Mind: Hitler, Hess, and the Analysts* (Oxford: Oxford University Press, 2014).

35. G. Ronald Hargreaves, "The Differential Aspects of the Psychoneuroses of War," in *The Neuroses of War*, ed. Emanuel Miller (London: Macmillan, 1940), 85–104.

36. Eugene B. Brody, "The World Federation for Mental Health: Its Origins and Contemporary Relevance to the WHO and WPA Policies," *World Psychiatry* 3,

no. 1 (2004): 54–55; George Brock Chisholm, "The Psychiatry of Enduring Peace and Social Progress," *Psychiatry* 9 (1946): 1–44. The journal was renamed *Psychiatry: Interpersonal and Biological Processes* in 1986, reflecting the epistemological change of psychiatric sciences.

37. WHO Archive, WHO4: Records of the Director General's Office.

38. Gerry Bowler, *Christmas in the Crosshairs: Two Thousand Years of Denouncing and Defending the World's Most Celebrated Holiday* (Oxford: Oxford University Press, 2016), 193.

39. George Brock Chisholm, *Can People Learn to Learn? How to Know Each Other* (New York: Harper, 1958).

40. Winfred Overholser, "Presidential Address," *American Journal of Psychiatry* 105, no. 1 (1948): 1–9.

41. William C. Menninger, "Presidential Address," *American Journal of Psychiatry* 106, no. 1 (1949): 4.

42. Ibid., 5.

43. Rebecca Jo Plant, "William Menninger's Campaign to Reform American Psychoanalysis, 1946–48," *History of Psychiatry* 16, no. 2 (2005): 181–202.

44. See Cornelia Navari, *Internationalism and the State in the Twentieth Century* (New York: Routledge, 2000).

45. WHO Archive, M4/445/2 J1.

46. Ibid., p. 1.

47. Ibid., p. 2.

48. W. G. Jilek, "Emil Kraepelin and Comparative Sociocultural Psychiatry," *European Archives of Psychiatry and Clinical Neuroscience* 245, no. 4–5 (1995): 231–238; Paul Hoff, "The Kraepelinian Tradition," *Dialogues in Clinical Neuroscience* 17, no. 1 (March 2015): 31–41.

49. Anne Harrington, *Mind Fixers: Psychiatry's Troubled Search for the Biology of Mental Illness* (New York: W. W. Norton, 2019).

50. German E. Berrios and R. Hauser, "The Early Development of Kraepelin's Ideas on Classification: A Conceptual History," *Psychological Medicine* 18 (1988): 813–821; Matthias M. Weber and Eric J. Engstrom, "Kraepelin's 'Diagnostic Cards': The Confluence of Clinical Research and Preconceived Categories," *History of Psychiatry* 8 (September 1997): 375–385.

51. G. R. Hargreaves, *Psychiatry and the Public Health* (London: Oxford University Press, 1958).

52. Siddiqi, *World Health and World Politics*, 41–47.

53. Article 55 of *The Charter of the United Nations* (San Francisco: United Nations, 1945), 11–12.

54. The Constitution was adopted by the International Health Conference held in New York from June 19 to July 22, 1946; it was signed on July 22, 1946, by the representatives of sixty-one states (*Official Records of the WHO*, no. 2 [June 1948]: 100), and entered into force on April 7, 1948. It has not been changed since its inauguration.

55. Farley, *Brock Chisholm*, 92.

56. See Amrith, *Decolonizing International Health*, 122. Also see Cueto, Brown, and Fee, "The Birth of the World Health Organization, 1945–1948," in *The World Health Organization*, 63–64.

57. Farley, *Brock Chisholm*, 53.

58. World Health Organization, *The First Ten Years of the World Health Organization* (Geneva: World Health Organization, 1958).

59. Siddiqi, *World Health and World Politics*.

60. The project was adjusted from "eradication" to "control" in the late 1960s. See Randall Packard, *A History of Global Health: Interventions into the Lives of Other Peoples* (Baltimore: Johns Hopkins University Press, 2016).

61. Cueto, Brown, and Fee, *The World Health Organization*, 66.

62. Wellcome Archives SA/BMA/B.87.

63. Representation of His Majesty's Government at the International Congress on Mental Health to be held in London in 1948, J. Lindsey to Miss Murray, December 17, 1947, code 403, file 5577, National Archives FO 370/1411.

64. International Congress on Mental Health, London, August 1948, code 403, file 310, National Archives FO 370/1525.

65. See Jonathan Toms, "Political Dimensions of 'the Psychosocial': The 1948 International Congress on Mental Health and the Mental Hygiene Movement," *History of Human Sciences* 25, no. 5 (December 2012): 91–106, https://doi.org/10.1177/0952695112470044.

66. J. C. Flugel, E. Matilda Goldberg, Mary Cockett, and S. Clement Brown, *International Congress on Mental Health, London, 1948*, ed. John Carl Flügel, 4 vols. (New York: H. K. Lewis & Co. and Columbia University Press, 1948).

67. Brody, "The World Federation for Mental Health."

68. Peter Mandler, *Return from the Natives: How Margaret Mead Won the Second World War and Lost the Cold War* (New Haven: Yale University Press, 2013).

69. Margaret Mead, *Cultural Patterns and Technical Change (1)* (Dublin: Mentor Book, 1955), 5.

70. International Congress on Mental Health, *Mental Health and World Citizenship: A Statement Prepared for the International Congress on Mental Health: London, 1948* (London: World Federation for Mental Health, 1948), 47.

71. *Chronicle of the World Health Organization* 4, no. 1 (1950): 6.

72. Chisholm, *Can People Learn to Learn?*

73. World Health Organization, *WHO and Mental Health 1949–1961* (Geneva: World Health Organization, 1962).

74. Tsung-yi Lin, *Road to Psychiatry: Across the East and the West* (Taipei: Daw Shiang Publishing, 1994), 96–97.

75. After his training as a psychiatrist at Peking Union Medical College Hospital, Yü-Lin Ch'eng founded Nanjing Brain Hospital. After World War II, he went to Taiwan with the Chinese Nationalist (Kuomintang) government and briefly served as the first superintendent of Taiwan Provincial Mental Hospital before he relocated to Michigan, USA.

76. See United Nations Economic and Social Council, "Economics and Social Council Official Records: Third Year, Seventh Session, Supplement No. 8; Report of the Social Commission" (1948), 28, 29.

77. Lucien Bovet, *Psychiatric Aspects of Juvenile Delinquency: A Study Prepared on Behalf of the World Health Organization as a Contribution to the United Nations Programme for the Prevention of Crime and Treatment of Offenders* (Geneva: World Health Organization, 1951).

78. WHO Archive, WHO/MHA/1, p. 2.

79. Wolfgang Rüdig, *Anti-nuclear Movements: A World Survey of Opposition to Nuclear Energy* (Harlow, UK: Longman, 1990), 54–55.

80. Executive Board, World Federation for Mental Health, Sub-Committee on Mental Health Aspects of Atomic Energy, Minutes of Second Meeting, New York, November 9, 1956, folder 620.992:3, in "Peaceful Use," UNESCO Archives, Paris.

81. WHO Archive, WHO/AH/AE/2.

82. WHO Archive, WHO/MH/AE/2.

83. Ran Zwigenberg, "Healing a Sick World: Psychiatric Medicine and the Atomic Age," *Medical History* 62, no. 1 (2017): 27–49.

84. WHO Archive, M4/445/2 J1, p. 3.

85. Considered the father of comparative psychiatry, Emil Kraepelin is most renowned for his phenomenology-based classification of psychiatric symptoms and

his work on comparative psychiatry. Regarding classification, he described dementia praecox and manic depression. See E. Kraepelin and G. M. Robertson, *Dementia Praecox and Paraphrenia* (Edinburgh: Livingstone, 1919); G. E. Berrios, R. Luque, and J. M. Villagran, "Schizophrenia: A Conceptual History," *International Journal of Psychology and Psychological Therapy* 3 (2003): 111–140. Kraepelin's work in comparative psychiatry was preceded by a series of travels, including to Indonesia and North America.

86. Hargreaves to Lemkau, September 8, 1954, WHO Archive, M4/445/2/J2.

87. See Karen Kruse Thomas, *Health and Humanity: A History of the Johns Hopkins Bloomberg School of Public Health, 1935–1985* (Baltimore: Johns Hopkins University Press, 2016).

88. Lemkau to Hargreaves, May 30, 1954, WHO Archive, M4/445/2 J2.

89. Landis to Hargreaves, April 15, 1953, WHO Archive, M4/445/2 J1.

90. Hargreaves to Landis, June 17, 1953, WHO Archive, M4/445/2 J1.

91. WHO Archive, M4/445/2 J1.

92. Paul Victor Lemkau, *Mental Hygiene in Public Health*, 2d ed. (New York: McGraw-Hill, 1955). In the book he offered two types of preparatory work in preventive psychiatry: being prepared to meet generalized and unpredictable stresses, and being prepared to meet expected stresses.

93. Hargreaves to Lemkau, October 7, 1953, WHO Archive, M4/445/2/ J1.

94. Lemkau to Hargreaves, May 12, 1954, WHO Archive, M4/445/2 J2.

95. WHO Archive, M4/445/2 J1.

96. See Clyde Kiser et al., "The World of the Milbank Memrorial Fund in Population since 1928," *Milbank Memorial Fund Quarterly* 49, no. 4 (1971): 15–66; Clyde Kiser, "The Role of the Milbank Memorial Fund in the Early History of the Association," *Population Index* 47, no. 3 (1981): 490–494.

97. Hargreaves to Gruenberg, July 22, 1955, WHO Archive, M4/445/2 J2.

98. Ernest M. Gruenberg, "The Epidemiology of Mental Disease," *Scientific American* 190, no. 3 (1954): 38–42. In the article, Gruenberg laments that Adolf Meyer's work on the relationship between social conditions and mental illness in the 1930s had gone uncompleted.

99. Dorothy Porter and UC Medical Humanities Consortium, *Health Citizenship: Essays in Social Medicine and Biomedical Politics* (Berkeley: University of California Medical Humanities Press, 2011).

100. London School of Tropical Hygiene and Medicine Archives, ACC/OS.

101. WHO Archive, WHO/MENT/178.

102. WHO Archive, M4/445/2, Paul Lemkau.

103. WHO Archive, M4/445/2 J4.

104. Boudreau to Peterson, October 10, 1957, WHO Archive, M4/445/2 J5.

105. The philosophy of why epidemiology is assumed to illustrate the reason of cause is beyond the scope of this book.

106. WHO Archive, M4/445/2 J5.

107. Ibid.

108. For example, see Marvin K. Opler's monograph, *Culture, Psychiatry and Human Values: The Method and Values of a Social Psychiatry* (Springfield, IL: C. C. Thomas, 1956), which also gave some insights into the emerging project.

109. Howard Higginbotham, *Third World Challenge to Psychiatry: Culture Accommodation and Mental Health Care* (Honolulu: East-West Center by the University of Hawaii Press, 1984).

110. Marvin K. Opler, "Schizophrenia and Culture," *Scientific American* 197, no. 2 (1957): 110.

111. This section also marked World War II as a watershed era in psychiatry. In the newsletter, Wittkower et al. wrote, "In the years since World War II psychiatrists and social scientists on every continent have begun to tackle problems whose solutions are recognized to be linked to research going beyond national and cultural boundaries. Whole populations in Asia, Africa and South America are rapidly undergoing fundamental transformations in their mode of life. People are shifting and moving, social and economic structures are rapidly changing, technologically backward populations are being drawn out of relative isolation into the complex fabric of modern industrial economies. The conflict of competing socio-political and ideological systems has given this second half of the twentieth century an air of unrest and crisis." See E. D. Wittkower, F. Jacob, and F. D. Pande, editorial in *Newsletter of Transcultural Research in Mental Health Problems* (Department of Psychiatry and Department of Sociology and Anthropology, McGill University), no. 1 (February 1956).

112. E. D. Wittkower, F. Jacob, and F. D. Pande, *Newsletter of Transcultural Research in Mental Health Problems*, no. 2 (1956).

113. Wittkower to Candau, July 8, 1956, WHO Archive, M4/445/2 J3.

114. WHO Archive, M4/445/2 J3.

115. Ibid.

116. Ibid.

117. J. Bains, "Race, Culture and Psychiatry: A History of Transcultural Psychiatry," *History of Psychiatry* 16, no. 2 (2005): 139–154.

118. Peter Mandler, "One World, Many Cultures: Margaret Mead and the Limits to Cold War Anthropology," *History Workshop Journal*, no. 68 (2009): 150–172.

119. See the discussion in chapter 5 below.

120. World Federation for Mental Health, *Cultural Patterns and Technical Change: A Manual* (Paris: UNESCO, 1953), 348.

121. Mandler, *Return from the Natives*, 267.

122. Wittkower, Jacob, and Pande, editorial.

123. Comments from Paul Lemkau, *Newsletter of Transcultural Research in Mental Health Problems*, no. 3 (December 1957); Wittkower, Jacob, and Pande, editorial.

124. See Menry B. M. Murphy, "Cultural Factors in the Mental Health of Malayan Students," in Daniel Funkenstein, ed., *The Student and Mental Health: An International View* (Cambridge, MA: Riverside Press, 1959). In Murphy's own words, the principles are:

(1) In transcultural psychiatry observations will usually be more useful and meaningful when framed in comparative terms than if left vague or related to abstract standards. (The Malay show little schizophrenia ... than what?)
(2) Where comparisons are offered, the groups or data being compared should be explicitly defined, not simply implied.
(3) Where comparisons are offered, care should also be taken to ensure that the data or situations are comparable.
(4) Reference to cultural traits should as far as possible be in terms of specific behavior patterns, and value judgement should be preferably avoided.
(5) The means by which information are obtained.

125. Vincenzo F. Di Nicola, "Memory and Appreciation: Henry MB Murphy MD PhD, 1915–1987," *Canadian Journal of Psychiatry* 33, no. 5 (1988): 424.

126. Henry B. M. Murphy, *Comparative Psychiatry: The International and Intercultural Distribution of Mental Illness* (Berlin: Springer-Verlag, 1982).

127. Giovanni de Girolamo and Norman Sartorius, eds., *Promoting Mental Health Internationally* (London: Gaskell, 1999).

128. Norman Sartorius and John Talbott, "International Mental Health Advocacy Organizations: An Interview with Norman Sartorius," *Journal of Nervous and Mental Disease* 199, no. 8 (2011): 557–561.

129. Theodore Brown, "'Stress' in US Wartime Psychiatry: World War II and the Immediate Aftermath," in *Stress, Shock, and Adaptation in the Twentieth Century*, ed. David Cantor and Edmund Ramsden (Rochester, NY: University of Rochester Press, 2014), 121–141.

Chapter 3

1. Anne M. Lovell, "The World Health Organization and the Contested Beginnings of Psychiatry Epidemiology as an International Discipline: One Rope, Many Strands," *International Journal of Epidemiology* 43, suppl. 1 (2014): 16–18.

2. The First WHO Seminar on Psychiatric Diagnosis, Classification, and Statistics, Alan Mason Chesney Medical Archives, PA/66.109.

3. NIMH, WZ 290 K16C 1964.

4. NIMH, W6 P3 v5772.

5. For example, in 1888, an international classification of mental diseases was proposed by Walther Channing.

6. E. Stengel, "Classification of Mental Disorders," *Bulletin of the World Health Organization* 21, no. 4–5 (1959): 601–663.

7. Ibid., 602.

8. Matthew Smith, "A Fine Balance: Individualism, Society and the Prevention of Mental Illness in the United States, 1945–1968," *Palgrave Communications* 2 (2016), article number 16024, DOI: 10.1057/palcomms.2016.24.

9. Ernest M. Gruenberg, "The Epidemiology of Mental Disease," *Scientific American* 190, no. 3 (1954): 38–42.

10. Erich Fromm, *The Heart of Man: Its Genius for Good and Evil* (London: Routledge & Kegan Paul, 1965).

11. Cited in Martin Birnbach, *Neo-Freudian Social Philosophy* (Stanford, CA: Stanford University Press, 1961).

12. See Randall Packard, *A History of Global Health: Interventions into the Lives of Other Peoples* (Baltimore: Johns Hopkins University Press, 2016). Packard does not mention noninfectious diseases when he explains the expansion of the social sciences.

13. Nancy Campbell, "The Spirit of St. Louis: The Contributions of Lee N. Robins to North American Psychiatric Epidemiology," *International Journal of Epidemiology* 43, suppl. 1 (2013): 19–28.

14. John Farley, "The Interim Commission, 1946–48: The Long Wait," in *Brock Chisholm, the World Health Organization, and the Cold War* (Vancouver: University of British Columbia Press, 2008), 48–57.

15. Eduardo Krapf, "Preliminary Statement on a Research Project Dealing with Mental Health and Diseases from a Comparative Point of View," February 22, 1953, WHO Archive, M4/445/2.

16. Julian Leff, personal communication with the author, London, 2010.

17. Gillespie to Edward Mopather (date before March 30, 1939), IOP/PP3/4/7/2. Gillespie continued: "Knowledge of the best means of protecting [a civilian] himself, and those who are dependent on him, is also important. But the first consideration is by far the greater. Previous personal preparation of a more general kind, calculated to appeal to the idealism of the individual citizen, is also greatly to be desired. As an adjuvant to this, the motive of any kind of personal gain should be completely removed from war, so that people may not be disturbed in their courage either by the presence of this motive in themselves, or by witnessing its operation in others. Those known to have been psychiatric casualties in the last war, especially pensioners, should be evacuated beforehand from the dangerous areas."

18. Aubrey Lewis Papers, IOP/PP3/5/6 (April 15, 1943). Before World War II, a committee called the Study of International Psychology had been organized at IOP in the hope that it would yet be possible to understand and mitigate the psychological forces leading to war. Committee members believed that they were called to mitigate war's evil effects. Some psychologists felt that this could best be accomplished by increasing the efficiency of the government's military actions against the Nazis, while others preferred to provide help to civilian populations. This committee, however, was less influential than military psychiatrists. See Pryns Hopkins to Edward Mapother, September 29, 1938, IOP/PP3/4/2/3.

19. Aubrey Lewis Papers, IOP/PP3/5/6 (April 15, 1943).

20. Aubrey Lewis Papers, IOP/PP3/5/26 (1959), p. 1.

21. Aubrey Lewis Papers, IOP/PP3/5/26 (1959).

22. In the meantime, the Mental Health Unit of the WHO was also reconsidering the custodial functions of mental health hospitals.

23. Traolach S. Brugha, Lorna Wing, John Cooper, and Norman Sartorius, "Contribution and Legacy of John Wing, 1923–2010," *British Journal of Psychiatry* 198, no. 3 (March 2011): 176–178, https://doi.org/10.1192/bjp.bp.110.084889.

24. Erving Goffman, *Asylums: Essays on the Social Situation of Mental Patients and Other Inmates* (Harmondsworth, UK: Penguin Books, 1968).

25. Ibid.

26. J. K. Wing and George William Brown, *Institutionalism and Schizophrenia: A Comparative Study of Three Mental Hospitals, 1960–1968* (Cambridge: Cambridge University Press, 1970), 13.

27. Ibid.

28. Ibid.

29. J. K. Wing and Antha M. Hailey, *Evaluating a Community Psychiatric Service: The Camberwell Register, 1964–71* (London: Oxford University Press and Nuffield Provincial Hospitals Trust, 1972), 3–9.

30. Another famous survey study in Camberwell was carried out by sociologist George Brown and clinical psychologist Tirril Harris between 1969 and 1973 on the relationship between life stresses and depression. See Rhodri Hayward, "Sadness in Camberwell: Imagining Stress and Constructing History in Postwar Britain," in *Stress, Shock, and Adaptation in the Twentieth Century*, ed. David Cantor and Edmund Ramsden (Rochester, NY: University of Rochester Press, 2014), 320–342.

31. See chapter 2.

32. Andrew Scull, "The Mental Health Sector and the Social Sciences in Post-World War II USA; Part 1: Total War and Its Aftermath," *History of Psychiatry* 22, no. 1 (2011): 3–19.

33. For example, Robert Felix, speech delivered on February 6, 1946, at Menninger Foundation in Topeka, Kansas; and speech delivered on October 8, 1946, at the Annual Meeting of the Southern Psychiatric Association, Richmond, VA, Robert Felix personal papers, NIMH archive.

34. Karen Kruse Thomas, *Health and Humanity: A History of the Johns Hopkins Bloomberg School of Public Health, 1935–1985* (Baltimore: Johns Hopkins University Press, 2016).

35. E. John Cooper and Norman Sartorius, *A Companion to the Classification of Mental Disorders* (Oxford: Oxford University Press, 2013).

36. "The Effect of Urbanization on Mental Health," WPRO Report on Asia Family Conference in the Philippines, box 436833488, Alan Mason Chesney Medical Archives.

37. August B. Hollingshead and Frederick C. Redlich, "Social Stratification and Psychiatric Disorders," *American Sociological Review* 18, no. 2 (1953): 163–169. Their work later received the MacIver Award of the American Sociological Association.

38. Edmund Ramsden and Matthew Smith, "Remembering the West End: Social Science, Mental Health, and the American Urban Environment, 1939–1968," *Urban History* 45, no. 1 (2017): 128–149.

39. Leo Srole, Thomas S. Langner, Stanley T. Michael, Marvin K. Opler, and Thomas A. C. Rennie, *Mental Health in the Metropolis: The Midtown Manhattan Study* (New York: McGraw-Hill, 1962). Also see B. Pasamanick, "A Survey of Mental Disease in an Urban Population. IV. An Approach to Total Prevalence Rates," *Archives of General Psychiatry* 5, no. 2 (1961): 151–155.

40. See Robert Felix, "Research in Mental Health," speech at the Second Latin American Seminar on Mental Health, sponsored by the Pan American Health

Organization, World Health Organization, September 8–15, 1963, Buenos Aires, Argentina, Robert Felix personal papers, NIMH archive.

41. Joseph Zubin, "Cross-National Study of Diagnosis of the Mental Disorders: Methodology and Planning," *American Journal of Psychiatry* 125, no. 10S (1969): 12–20; E. John Cooper, Robert Kendell, Barry J. Gurland, Norman Sartorius, and Tibor Farkas, "Cross-National Study of Diagnosis of the Mental Disorders: Some Results from the First Comparative Investigation," *American Journal of Psychiatry* 125, no. 10 (1969): 21–29.

42. R. E. Kendell et al., "Diagnostic Criteria of American and British Psychiatrists," *Archives of General Psychiatry* 25, no. 2 (1971).

43. See Marcos Cueto, Theodore M. Brown, and Elizabeth Fee, *The World Health Organization: A History* (Cambridge: Cambridge University Press, 2019).

44. Morton Kramer, USSR trip concluding remarks, 1963, box 436833488, Alan Mason Chesney Medical Archives.

45. Benjamin Zajicek, "Soviet Psychiatry and the Origins of the Sluggish Schizophrenia Concept, 1912–1936," *History of the Human Sciences* 31, no. 2 (2018): 88–105, https://doi.org/10.1177/0952695117746057.

46. Report of Asia Family Conference in the Philippines, 1962, box 436833488, Alan Mason Chesney Medical Archives.

47. Julian P. Leff, *Psychiatry around the Globe: A Transcultural View*, 2nd ed. (London: Gaskell, 1988).

48. Tsung-yi Lin, *Road to Psychiatry: Across the East and the West* (Taipei: Daw Shiang Publishing, 1994), 93.

49. Tsung-yi Lin, "The Epidemiological Study of Mental Disorders by W.H.O.," *Social Psychiatry* 1, no. 4 (1967): 204–206.

50. See chapter 4.

51. WPRO, WHO Archive, M4/445/2.

52. Paul Sivadon, "The Development of a Science of Mental Health," presented at World Federation for Mental Health, 12th Meeting, Barcelona, 1959; quoted in Esther M. Thornton, *Planning and Action for Mental Health* (London: World Federation for Mental Health, 1961), 155–162.

53. Thornton, *Planning and Action for Mental Health*, 158.

54. Ibid., 160.

55. World Federation for Mental Health, *Cultural Patterns and Technical Change: A Manual* (Paris: UNESCO, 1953), 348.

56. Executive Board, World Federation for Mental Health, Sub-Committee on Mental Health Aspects of Atomic Energy, Minutes of Second Meeting, New York, November 9, 1956, folder 620.992:3, in "Peaceful Use," UNESCO Archives, Paris, 348.

57. According to Norman Sartorius, the WFMH did not ultimately contribute much to research apart from its achievement in the commemoration of 1961 as World Mental Health Year. N. Sartorius, personal communication with the author, Geneva, 2010. In the 1970s, its financial situation deteriorated until Lin's appointment as WFMH president. See Eugene B. Brody, "The World Federation for Mental Health: Its Origins and Contemporary Relevance to the WHO and WPA Policies," *World Psychiatry* 3, no. 1 (2004): 54–55.

58. Peter Mandler, *Return from the Natives: How Margaret Mead Won the Second World War and Lost the Cold War* (New Haven: Yale University Press, 2013), 267.

59. Lin, *Road to Psychiatry*, 116.

60. Kelley Lee, *The World Health Organization (WHO)* (Abington, UK: Routledge, 2008). See also Farley, "The Interim Commission, 1946–48," 48–57.

61. Lee, *The World Health Organization*, 134.

62. Lin, *Road to Psychiatry*, 118.

63. Tsung-yi Lin to the Director General, June 11, 1965, WHO Archive, M4/86/12.

64. Gian Luca Burci and Claude-Henri Vignes, *World Health Organization* (The Hague: Kluwer Law International, 2004), 195.

65. For a detailed explanation of postwar psychiatric culture in the United States, see Marijke Gijswijt-Hofstra, *Psychiatric Cultures Compared: Psychiatry and Mental Health Care in the Twentieth Century: Comparisons and Approaches* (Amsterdam: Amsterdam University Press, 2005), 456.

66. World Health Organization, Technical Report Series, 223 (1961).

67. *Chronicle of the World Health Organization* 16 (1962): 306–311.

68. World Health Organization, *The Second Ten Years of the World Health Organization* (Geneva: World Health Organization, 1968), xi.

69. Eileen Brooke, GB 0370 PP32, box 3, Queen Mary, University of London Library Archives.

70. Lovell, "The World Health Organization and the Contested Beginnings of Psychiatry Epidemiology," 16–18.

71. World Health Organization, "W.H.O. Mental Health News," *Mental Health Section* 1, no. 3 (1963).

72. Peter Baan to E. A. Babayan, May 4, 1965, WHO Archive, M4/87/7.

73. IOP/CAM9/2.

74. See "National Clearinghouse of Mental Health Information," *Schizophrenia Bulletin* 1, no. 3 (1970): 51–53.

75. In 1962, the meeting between Tsung-yi Lin and the NIMH experts was attended by Morton Kramer, J. Zubin, B. Pasamanick, S. Greenhouse, M. Katz, and Robert Felix. See Lin, *Road to Psychiatry*, 117.

76. Editor, "Conversation with Joy Moser," *British Journal of Addiction* 79 (1984): 355–363.

77. Discussion Groups at WFMH Annual Meeting, Bern, August 3–7, 1964, WHO Archive, M4/86/12.

78. In the same year, this method was employed by the London Group in establishing Camberwell Registers.

79. WHO Archive, M4/87/7.

80. WHO Archive, M4/87/7.

81. In 1963, the WFMH planned to relocate its headquarters from London to Geneva, not only because of the cheaper rent but also because of Geneva's international (cosmopolitan) environment. See WHO Archive, WFMH/Ex. 39/16.

82. For example, for the Moscow seminar, five participants were from the USSR, and others were from Bulgaria, Czechoslovakia, East Germany, Hungary, Poland, Romania, and Yugoslavia. WHO Archive, M4/440/23 (4) 1.

83. Michael Shepherd to Tsung-yi Lin, February 16, 1966, WHO Archive, M4/440/23 (65).

84. WHO Archive, M4/441/11.

85. For example, it was during Tsung-yi Lin's visit to Buenos Aires in 1964 that Argentinian doctor A. Bonhour's epidemiological research program came to Lin's attention. From the WHO Archive, M4/441/11.

86. WHO Archive, M4/87/7(66) J4.

87. John Cooper, "Towards a Common Language for Mental Health Workers," in *Promoting Mental Health Internationally*, ed. Giovanni De Girolamo and N. Sartorius (London: Gaskell, 1999), 14–46.

88. See Eric Stengel, "A Comparative Study of Psychiatric Classification," *Proceedings of the Royal Society of Medicine* 53, no. 2 (1960): 123–130.

89. For example, participants of the first meeting included the British experts Aubrey Lewis, Michael Shepherd, W. P. D. Logan from Maudsley Hospital, and Eileen Brooke from the Ministry of Health.

90. WHO Archive, M4/87/7.

91. Cooper, "Towards a Common Language for Mental Health Workers," 19.

92. M. Kramer, N. Sartorius, and A. Jablensky, "The ICD-9 Classification of Mental Disorders: A Review of Its Development and Contents," *Acta Psychiatrica Scandinavica*, no. 59 (1979): 241–262.

93. The qualifications were listed as follows: "(1) competence in the field of psychiatric diagnosis and classification and/or collection and analysis of psychiatric statistics; (2) representative of a school of psychiatry and acquainted with others, or having wide knowledge of biostatistical work in psychiatry; (3) influential in own country (if possible also more widely); (4) willingness to collaborate over a long period." WHO Archive, M4/87/7.

94. They were: "(1) schizophrenia; (2) the group of diseases included under the category of psychogenic reaction; (3) psychiatric disorders encountered in childhood; (4) mental subnormality (also known as retardation, defect, deficiency, etc.); (5) psychiatric disorders associated with senility and presenility; (6) pathological personality." WHO Archive, M4/87/7.

95. WHO Archive, M4/445/22 J3.

96. WHO Archive, M4/87(65) J3, 4.

97. WHO Archive, M4/87/7.

98. Ibid.

99. WHO Archive, M4/87/7(65) J4.

100. They include Argentina, Australia, Ceylon, Colombia, Denmark, France, India, Japan, Lebanon, Nigeria, Norway, Sudan, Switzerland, Taiwan (then China), Thailand, Turkey, the UK, the USA, and the USSR.

101. See World Health Organization, *Report of the International Pilot Study of Schizophrenia* (Geneva: World Health Organization, 1973); International Pilot Study of Schizophrenia and World Health Organization, *Schizophrenia: A Multinational Study; A Summary of the Initial Evaluation Phase of the International Pilot Study of Schizophrenia* (Geneva: World Health Organization, 1975).

102. WHO Archive, M4/87/7(65) J3.4.

103. WHO Archive, M4/87/7.

104. WHO Archive, M4/87/7(65) J3.4.

105. Tsung-yi Lin to E. Gruenberg, May 25, 1966, WHO Archive, M4/87/7 (66).

106. Cooper, "Towards a Common Language for Mental Health Workers," 23.

107. See World Health Organization, *Schizophrenia: An International Follow-up Study* (Chichester, UK: Wiley, 1979). To date, various arguments have been put forward about why prognoses of schizophrenic patients are better in developing countries. One of the most promising explanations is that in family-oriented societies, patients enjoy better support from family members. Recent studies, however, have pointed out the sample bias in the study. For example, see Alex Cohen, "Prognosis for Schizophrenia in the Third World: A Reevaluation of Cross-Cultural Research," *Culture, Medicine and Psychiatry* 16, no. 1 (1992): 53–75.

108. Norman Sartorius, A. Jablensky, and A. A. Korten, "Early Manifestations and First Contact Incidence of Schizophrenia in Different Cultures: A Preliminary Report on the Evaluative Phase of the WHO Collaborative Study on Determinants of Outcome of Severe Mental Disorders," *Psychological Medicine*, no. 16 (1986): 909–928; A. Jablensky et al., "Schizophrenia: Manifestations, Incidence and Course in Different Cultures: A World Health Organization 10-Country Study," *Psychological Medicine* 20, suppl. (1992).

109. Cooper, "Towards a Common Language for Mental Health Workers," table 2.2, 28.

110. For example, the WHO (then led by Norman Sartorius) embarked on the study of Standardized Assessment of Depressive Disorders (SADD) during the early 1980s. See Norman Sartorius and World Health Organization, *Depressive Disorders in Different Cultures: Report on the WHO Collaborative Study on Standardized Assessment of Depressive Disorders* (Geneva: World Health Organization, 1983).

111. See H. G. Hwu, C. C. Chen, J. S. Strauss, K. L. Tan, M. T. Tsuang, and W. S. Tseng, "A Comparative Study on Schizophrenia Diagnosed by ICD-9 and DSM-III: Course, Family History and Stability of Diagnosis," *Acta Psychiatrica Scandinavica* 77 (1988): 87–97.

112. G. C. Tooth to Peter Baan, July 26, 1965, WHO Archive, M4/440/23 (65) 3.

113. WHO Archive, M4/440/23(65).

114. G. C. Tooth to Peter Baan, October 1, 1965, WHO Archive, M4/440/23 (65).

115. M. G. Candau to Chief of Mental Health Unit, 1968, WHO Archive, M4/440/23 (4).

116. Ibid.

117. Peter Baan to J. E. Rochalskij, August 13, 1968, WHO Archive, M4/440/23 (4).

118. Kelley Lee, "Global Institutions: The World Health Organization (the WHO)," *Nursing Management* (Harrow) 18, no. 5 (September 1, 2011): 12; doi: 10.7748/nm.18.5.12.s2.

Chapter 4

1. Anthony V. S. De Reuck and Ruth Porter, *Transcultural Psychiatry* (London: Churchill, 1965), 22.

2. Ibid.

3. See chapter 3 on the qualification of experts.

4. Sheila Jasanoff and Sang-Hyun Kim, *Dreamscapes of Modernity: Sociotechnical Imaginaries and the Fabrication of Power* (Chicago: University of Chicago Press, 2015), 4.

5. Meticulous efforts to write the fifth chapter of the *International Classification of Diseases* (WHO, 1975) represent this mentality in modern psychiatry. The *ICD* system is used in 117 WHO member countries and is available in 43 languages to assist with reporting morbidity and mortality data. Moreover, the *ICD* system has become the primary indicator of health status in use among all WHO members. This system was the outcome of the *ICD* authors' original objective of providing all-encompassing diagnoses for mental disorders.

6. See Waltraud Ernst, *Mad Tales from the Raj: The European Insane in British India, 1800–1858* (London: Routledge, 1991); Jock McCulloch, *Colonial Psychiatry and "The African Mind"* (Cambridge: Cambridge University Press, 1995); Megan Vaughan, *Curing Their Ills: Colonial Power and African Illness* (Cambridge, UK: Polity, 1991); Sloan Mahone and Megan Vaughan, *Psychiatry and Empire* (Basingstoke, UK: Palgrave Macmillan, 2007); Yu-Chuan Wu, "Disappearing Anger: Fujisawa Shigeru's Psychological Experiments on Formosan Aborigines in the Late Colonial Period," *East Asian Science, Technology and Society* 6, no. 2 (2012): 199–219.

7. In the case of Japan, see Janice Matsumura, "State Propaganda and Mental Disorders: The Issue of Psychiatric Casualties among Japanese Soldiers during the Asia-Pacific War," *Bulletin of the History of Medicine* 78, no. 4 (2004): 804–835; Ran Zwigenberg, *Hiroshima: The Origins of Global Memory Culture* (Cambridge: Cambridge University Press, 2014).

8. Javed Siddiqi, *World Health and World Politics: The World Health Organization and the UN System* (Columbia: University of South Carolina Press, 1995).

9. Anne-Emanuelle Birn, *Marriage of Convenience: Rockefeller International Health and Revolutionary Mexico* (Rochester, NY: University of Rochester Press, 2006).

10. Peter Galison, *Image and Logic: A Material Culture of Microphysics* (Chicago: University of Chicago Press, 1997).

11. According to Galison, trading partners can hammer out a plan for local coordination, despite vast global differences. In an even more sophisticated way, cultures in interaction frequently establish contact languages, systems of discourse that can vary from the most function-specific jargon to semispecific pidgins to full-fledged

creoles rich enough to support activities as complex as poetry and metalinguistic reflection. Galison, *Image and Logic*, 783.

12. Randall Packard, *A History of Global Health: Interventions into the Lives of Other Peoples* (Baltimore: Johns Hopkins University Press, 2016).

13. Harry Collins, *Are We All Scientific Experts Now?* (Cambridge: Polity, 2014).

14. John Krige, ed., *How Knowledge Moves: Writing the Transnational History of Science and Technology* (Chicago: University of Chicago Press, 2019), 17

15. Sunil Amrith, *Decolonizing International Health: India and Southeast Asia, 1930–1965* (New York: Palgrave Macmillan, 2006). For a postcolonial critique within global health, see Warwick Anderson, "Making Global Health History: The Postcolonial Worldliness of Biomedicine," *Social History of Medicine* 27, no. 2 (2014): 377–378. For self-fashioning among Southeast Asian scientists, see Warwick Anderson and Han Pols, "Scientific Patriotism: Medical Science and National Self-Fashioning in Southeast Asia," *Comparative Studies in Society and History* 54, no. 1 (2012): 93–113.

16. Jasanoff and Kim, *Dreamscapes of Modernity*.

17. Marcos Cueto, Theodore M. Brown, and Elizabeth Fee, *The World Health Organization: A History* (Cambridge: Cambridge University Press, 2019), 77. Also see Jessica Lynne Pearson, *The Colonial Politics of Global Health: France and the United Nations in Postwar Africa* (Cambridge, MA: Harvard University Press, 2018).

18. Anne M. Lovell, "The World Health Organization and the Contested Beginnings of Psychiatry Epidemiology as an International Discipline: One Rope, Many Strands," *International Journal of Epidemiology* 43, suppl. 1 (2014): 16–18.

19. See McCulloch, *Colonial Psychiatry and "the African Mind."*

20. John C. Carothers, *The African Mind in Health and Disease: A Study in Ethnopsychiatry* (Geneva: World Health Organization, 1953).

21. Lovell, "The World Health Organization and the Contested Beginnings of Psychiatry Epidemiology."

22. See Yolana Pringle, "Investigating 'Mass Hysteria' in Early Postcolonial Uganda: Benjamin H. Kagwa, East African Psychiatry, and the Gisu," *Journal of the History of Medicine and Allied Sciences* 70, no. 1 (2015): 105–136.

23. H. J. Simons, "Mental Disease in Africa: Racial Determinisms," *Journal of Mental Science* 104, no. 135 (1958): 377–388.

24. WHO Archive, M4/445/2/AFRO.

25. Matthew Heaton, "The Politics and Practice of Thomas Adeoye Lambo: Towards a Post-colonial History of Transcultural Psychiatry," *History of Psychiatry* 29, no. 3 (March 1, 2018): 315–330, doi: 10.1177/0957154X18765422.

26. T. A. Lambo, "The Role of Cultural Factors in Paranoid Psychosis among the Yoruba Tribe," *British Journal of Psychiatry* 101, no. 423 (1955): 239–266.

27. Heaton, "The Politics and Practice of Thomas Adeoye Lambo," 315–330.

28. Matthew Heaton, *Black Skin, White Coats: Nigerian Psychiatrists, Decolonization, and the Globalization of Psychiatry* (Athens: Ohio University Press, 2013).

29. Alexander H. Leighton, T. Adeoye Lambo, Charles C. Hughes, Dorothea C. Leighton, Jane M. Murphy, and David B. Macklin, *Psychiatric Disorder among the Yoruba* (Ithaca, NY: Cornell University Press, 1963).

30. Ibid.

31. Oye Gureje et al., "Mental Disorders among Adult Nigerians: Risks, Prevalence, and Treatment," in *The WHO Mental Health Surveys: Global Perspectives on the Epidemiology of Mental Disorders*, ed. Ronald C. Kessler and T. Bedirhan Ustun (Cambridge: Cambridge University Press, 2008), 211–237.

32. Mariano Ben Plotkin, ed., *Argentina on the Couch: Psychiatry, State, and Society, 1880 to the Present* (Albuquerque: University of New Mexico Press, 2003).

33. G. R. Hargreaves, *Psychiatry and the Public Health* (London: Oxford University Press, 1958).

34. WHO Archive, M4/445/2; Hugo Vezzetti, "From the Psychiatric Hospital to the Street: Enrique Pichon Riviere and the Diffusion of Psychoanalysis in Argentina," in Plotkin, *Argentina on the Couch*.

35. Cecilia Taiana, "Transatlantic Migration of the Disciplines of the Mind: Examination of the Reception of the Wundt's and Freud's Theories in Argentina," in *Internationalizing the History of Psychology*, ed. Adrian C. Brock (New York: New York University Press, 2009), 34–55.

36. Humberto Rotondo, Javier Mariategui, Pedro Aliaga, and Carlos Garcia-Pacheco, "Un estudio PS salud mental de la colectividad rural de Pachacamac" (A study of mental health in the rural community of Pachacamac), *Archivos de Criminologia, Neuro-Psiquiatria y Disciplinas Conexas* (Lima, Peru), n.s., 8, no. 31 (July-September 1960): 458–491.

37. Jehan Vellard, "The Concept of Soul and Illness among the American Indians," *Bulletin de l'Institut Français d'Études Andines* (Lima) 1 (1957–1958): 5–54.

38. See "Mental Health in Latin America," *Chronicle of the World Health Organization* 18 (1964), 328–334.

39. See Roberto Perdomo, "Premio vida y obra al servicio de la psiquiatria," *Revista Colombiana de Psiquiatría* 25, no. 4 (1996): 298–301. Heath was infamous for his involvement in CIA-sponsored psychiatric experiments as well as gay conversion

therapy. For an example of his work, see Robert G. Heath, "Pleasure and Brain Activity in Man," *Journal of Nervous and Mental Disease* 154, no. 1 (1972): 3–18.

40. Carlos A. León, "Fright: Its Psychiatric Implications," presented at the second Latin American Congress of Psychiatry, Mexico, November 1962.

41. Pierre Buekens, "From Hygiene and Tropical Medicine to Global Health," *American Journal of Epidemiology* 176, suppl. 7 (October 1, 2012): S1–S3.

42. See Kim Hopper, Glynn Harrison, Aleksandar Janca, and Norman Sartorius, *Recovery from Schizophrenia: An International Perspective* (Oxford: Oxford University Press, 2007), 86–99.

43. See World Health Organization, *Results of the Initial Evaluation Phase*, vol. I of *Report of the International Pilot Study of Schizophrenia* (Geneva: World Health Organization, 1973), 55.

44. The paper was Tsung-yi Lin, "A Study of the Incidence of Mental Disorder in Chinese and Other Cultures," *Psychiatry*, no. 15 (1953): 313–336.

45. Tsung-yi Lin, *Road to Psychiatry: Across the East and the West* (Taipei: Daw Shiang Publishing, 1994); Lin, "A Study of the Incidence of Mental Disorder in Chinese and Other Cultures."

46. Julian P. Leff, "Knocking on Doors of Asia," in *Psychiatry around the Globe: A Transcultural View*, 2nd ed. (London: Gaskell, 1988), 92–100. This account is among the few comprehensive analyses that neither overemphasizes nor overlooks these studies.

47. The principle was predominantly propagated by the UN Educational, Scientific, and Cultural Organization (UNESCO).

48. Barkan also mentions that race typology as an element of causal cultural explanation became largely discredited among the principal scientific communities in the United States and the United Kingdom before the end of World War II and that racial differentiation became restricted to physical characteristics. Moreover, prejudicial actions based on racial discrimination were deemed inappropriate during this time period. See Elazar Barkan, *The Retreat of Scientific Racism: Changing Concepts of Race in Britain and the United States between the World Wars* (Cambridge: Cambridge University Press, 1992).

49. The United Nations and its specialized agencies promoted the context of internationalism; hence, UNESCO took a leading role in fulfilling the initiatives through a series of programs. Intense debates on the relevance of race remained unresolved despite two ardent statements of intention, in 1950 and 1952, to reduce the role of race in science. UNESCO stated that no race is inferior or superior to another, and moreover, mental characteristics and personality traits have no place in racial categorization. Races are defined in scientific research merely as "populations."

Hargreaves provided a stark proclamation that the entire world is a single race, using the rhetoric of world citizenship, and proposed a manageable project to study the determinants of mental disorders comparatively in various countries. His proposal was greatly disparaged, however, particularly by a group representing transcultural psychiatry. See Jenny Reardon, *Race to the Finish: Identity and Governance in an Age of Genomics* (Princeton, NJ: Princeton University Press, 2004).

50. Lin, *Road to Psychiatry*.

51. Ibid. See also Michael Shiyung Liu, *Prescribing Colonization: The Role of Medical Practices and Policies in Japan-Ruled Taiwan, 1895–1945* (Ann Arbor, MI: Association for Asian Studies, 2009).

52. For example, see Yu-Chuan Wu and Hui-Wen Teng, "Tropics, Neurasthenia, and Japanese Colonizers: The Psychiatric Discourses in Late Colonial Taiwan," *Taiwan: A Radical Quarterly in Social Studies*, no. 54 (2004): 61–103.

53. For Africa and South Asia, see Mahone and Vaughan, *Psychiatry and Empire*. For Japanese colonies, Prasenjit Duara revealed the complexity of the human sciences in East Asia, which cannot be completely characterized by using English terms such as "anthropology" or "ethnography." In Japanese, *jinruigaku* means "the study of humankind." The word *minzoku*, which appeared later in the course of Japanese colonization, indicates the overlapping of race and culture.

54. Akira Hashimoto, "A 'German World' Shared among Doctors: A History of the Relationship between Japanese and German Psychiatry before World War II," *History of Psychiatry* 24, no. 2 (2013): 180–195.

55. Harry Yi-Jui Wu, "Tropical Stupor? An Investigation into Patients Affected by Earthquake and Tropical Weather in Colonial Taiwan," in *Trauma in History: Asian Perspectives*, ed. Mark S. Micale and Hans Pols (Cambridge: Cambridge University Press, forthcoming).

56. Ibid.

57. See Wei-Chi Chen, *Ino Kanori and the Emergence of Historical Ethnography in Taiwan* (Taipei: National Taiwan University Press, 2014).

58. Hiroshi Utena and Shin-Ichi Niwa, "The History of Schizophrenia Research in Japan," *Schizophrenia Bulletin* 18, no. 1 (1992): 67–73.

59. Akihito Suzuki, "Psychiatry of a Population: An Overview of the Imperial Themes in Japanese Psychiatry from the 1930s to the 1950s," the Tenth Japan at Chicago Conference: Medicine, Politics, and Culture in the Japanese Empire, May 11–12, 2012, conference proceedings, https://lucian.uchicago.edu/blogs/medicineandempire/sample-page/.

60. Yushi Uchimura, Haruko Akimoto, and Toshimi Ishibashi, "The Syndrome of Imu in the Ainu Race," *American Journal of Psychiatry*, no. 94 (1938): 1467–1469.

61. See Marnie Copland, *A Lin Odyssey* (New Orleans: Paraclete Press, 1987), 36; Dugald Christie, *Thirty Years in Moukden, 1883–1913: Being the Experiences and Recollections of Dugald Christie, C. M. G.* (1914; repr., London: Forgotten Books, 2017); Herbert Day Lamson, *Social Pathology in China* (Shanghai: Commercial Books, 1934).

62. Huiyu Cai, "Shaping Administration in Colonial Taiwan," in *Taiwan under Japanese Colonial Rules, 1895–1945*, ed. Ping-Hui Liao and David Der-wei Wang (New York: Columbia University Press, 2009), 97–121. Also see Liu, *Prescribing Colonization.*

63. Hsien Rin, "An Investigation into the Incidence and Clinical Symptoms of Mental Disorders among Formosan Aborigines," *Psychiatria et Neurologia Japonica* 63, no. 5 (1961): 480–500.

64. The report listed three main factors contributing to the identification of mental illness cases among aborigines. First, the community leaders' intimate knowledge of the residents facilitated an understanding of the personal lives of each person in the small villages. Second, the team found a complete absence of stigma attached to mental illness. Third, villagers possessed relatively uniform concepts of mental illness and healthy behavior.

65. Lin, "A Study of the Incidence of Mental Disorder in Chinese and Other Cultures."

66. Ming-cheng Miriam Lo, *Doctors within Borders: Profession, Ethnicity, and Modernity in Colonial Taiwan* (Berkeley: University of California Press, 2002).

67. Lin, *Road to Psychiatry*, 10.

68. Hsiu-Jung Chang, *The Medical School of National Taiwan University 1945–1950* (Taipei: National Taiwan University Press, 2013).

69. Lin, *Road to Psychiatry*, 23.

70. Ibid., 21.

71. Chr Rasch, "On the Influence of Tropical Climate on [the] Nervous System," *Journal of Taiwan Medical Affairs* (April 18, 1899).

72. See Uchimura, Akimoto, and Ishibashi, "The Syndrome of Imu in the Ainu Race." Also see Hsien Rin, "A Study of the Etiology of Koro in Respect to the Chinese Concept of Illness," *Journal of Psychiatry*, no. 11 (1965): 7–13. In addition to these findings, cases of frigophobia were reported in the 1970s by Y. H. Chang, H. Rin, and C. C. Chen, "Frigophobia: A Report of Five Cases," *Bulletin of the Chinese Society of Neurology and Psychiatry* 1, no. 2 (1975): 13. (Rin subsequently left epidemiology to pursue cultural psychiatry.) Patients in the reported observations suffered from an extreme morbid fear of cold. They wore heavy clothing when arriving at the hospital. The clothing typically covered areas of the body that are considered weak in classic Chinese thought on health. Patients were characterized as overprotective mothers and exhibited dependent personalities. Chang et al. explained that these symptoms were closely related to the traditional Chinese concepts of vitality and

the yin-yang principle. Moreover, the symptoms may have developed as regressive psychopathology, which is a displaced, symbolic manifestation of fear caused by threats to the patient's security and consequent imagining of death.

73. Shao-hsing Chen, "Taiwan as a Laboratory for the Study of Chinese Society and Culture," *Bulletin of the Institute of Ethnology Academia Sinica* 14 (1966): 1–14.

74. John Farley, *Brock Chisholm, the World Health Organization, and the Cold War* (Vancouver: University of British Columbia Press, 2008), 90.

75. Yi-Ping Lin and Shiyung Liu, "A Forgotten War: Malaria Eradication in Taiwan, 1905–65," in *Health and Hygiene in Chinese East Asia*, ed. Angela Leung (Durham: Duke University Press, 2011), 183–203.

76. Sunil S. Amrith, *Decolonizing International Health: India and Southeast Asia, 1930–65* (Basingstoke, UK: Palgrave Macmillan, 2006).

77. Anderson and Pols, "Scientific Patriotism."

78. Jasanoff and Kim, *Dreamscapes of Modernity*.

79. Galison, *Image and Logic*, 783.

80. John Cooper, "Towards a Common Language for Mental Health Workers," in *Promoting Mental Health Internationally*, ed. Giovanni De Girolamo and N. Sartorius (London: Gaskell, 1999), 14–46.

81. See Richard Lane, "Norman Sartorius: Psychiatry's Living Legend," *Lancet Psychiatry* 6, no. 10 (2019): 811–812. On the development of social psychiatry in Yugoslavia, see Mat Savelli, "Beyond Ideological Platitudes: Socialism and Psychiatry in Eastern Europe," *Palgrave Communications* 4 (2018): 45, doi: 10.1057/s41599-018-0100-1.

Chapter 5

1. See Andrew Scull, *Madness in Civilization: A Cultural History of Insanity from the Bible to Freud, from the Madhouse to Modern Medicine* (Princeton, NJ: Princeton University Press, 2015).

2. Randall Packard, *A History of Global Health: Interventions into the Lives of Other Peoples* (Baltimore: Johns Hopkins University Press, 2016), 128

3. E. Wittkower [with assistance of Hsien Rin], "Recent Developments in Transcultural Psychiatry," in *Transcultural Psychiatry: A Ciba Foundation Symposium*, ed. A. V. S. de Reuck and Ruth Porter (London: J & A Churchill, 1965), 4–25, doi: 10.1002/9780470719428.

4. See, for example, Charles Coulston Gillispie, *Science and Polity in France: The Revolutionary and Napoleonic Years* (Princeton, NJ: Princeton University Press, 2004); Michael D. Gordin, "Hegemonic Languages and Science," *Isis* 108, no. 3 (September 2017): 606–611; Kristine C. Harper, *Weather by the Numbers: The Genesis of Modern Meteorology* (Cambridge, MA: MIT Press, 2008).

5. Michael Ward, *Quantifying the World: UN Ideas and Statistics* (Bloomington: Indiana University Press, 2004).

6. Examples are mostly about infectious diseases.

7. WHO Archive, M4/445/2(c).

8. World Health Organization and Interim Commission, Minutes of the third session of the Interim Commission held in Geneva from March 31 to April 12, 1947, *Official Records of the World Health Organization*, no. 5.

9. Geoffrey C. Bowker and Susan Leigh Star, *Sorting Things Out: Classification and Its Consequences* (Cambridge, MA: MIT Press, 1999).

10. WHO Archive, M4/445/2(4).

11. Aubrey Lewis personal papers, Bethlem Archive.

12. J. de Ajuriaguerra to Lin, March 26, 1969, Aubrey Lewis personal papers, Bethlem archive.

13. 7 Montrose Court, Hill Turrets Close, Sheffield S11 9RF, to Tsung-yi Lin, April 29, 1969, Aubrey Lewis personal papers, Bethlem Archive.

14. Daniel Sledge, *Health Divided: Public Health and Individual Medicine in the Making of the Modern American State* (Lawrence: University of Kansas Press, 2017).

15. Anton A. Huurdeman, *The Worldwide History of Telecommunications* (New York: J. Wiley, 2003).

16. See Richard E. Luria and Paul R. McHugh, "Reliability and Clinical Utility of the Wing Present State Examination," *Archives of General Psychiatry* 30, no. 6 (1974): 866–871.

17. WHO Archive, M4/87/7(65) J4; John Wing to Tsung-yi Lin, June 21, 1966, WHO Archive, M4/87/7(66) J3.

18. WHO Archive, M4/445/22 J4.

19. Lorraine Daston and Peter Galison, *Objectivity* (New York: Zone Books, 2007).

20. WHO Archive, M4/445/22 J3.

21. Ibid.

22. WHO Archive, M4/440/23 (67).

23. WHO Archive, M4/440/23 (3) 5, 6.

24. Interlingua, developed between 1937 and 1951 by the International Auxiliary Language Association (IALA), is assumed to be the second or third most widely used international auxiliary language (IAL), after Esperanto and Ido, and the most widely used naturalistic IAL. See www.interlingua.com.

25. WHO Archive, M4/440/23 (65).

26. John Cooper, "Towards a Common Language for Mental Health Workers," in *Promoting Mental Health Internationally*, ed. Giovanni De Girolamo and N. Sartorius (London: Gaskell, 1999), 14–46.

27. World Health Organization, *Report of the International Pilot Study of Schizophrenia* (Geneva: World Health Organization, 1973), vol. 1, 90.

28. Lyman C. Wynne to Tsung-yi Lin, May 19, 1967, WHO Archive, M4/445/22 J5.

29. Comments on Research Schedules, WHO Archive, M4/445/22 J7.

30. Lyman C. Wynne to Tsung-yi Lin, March 28, 1967, WHO Archive, M4/445/22 J5.

31. Lyman C. Wynne to Tsung-yi Lin, February 27, 1967, WHO Archive, M4/445/22/ J4.

32. Wynne to Lin, May 19, 1967.

33. Soong, personal communication with author, Chiayi City, 2011. Chu-Chang Chen, personal communication with author, Taipei, 2011.

34. Norman Sartorius and John Talbott, "International Mental Health Advocacy Organizations: An Interview with Norman Sartorius," *Journal of Nervous and Mental Disease* 199, no. 8 (2011): 557–561.

35. Tsung-yi Lin, *Road to Psychiatry: Across the East and the West* (Taipei: Daw Shiang Publishing, 1994), 125; Cooper, "Towards a Common Language for Mental Health Workers," 113–159.

36. Erik Ströngren to Tsung-yi Lin, September 30, 1966, WHO Archive, M4/87/ (66), J4.

37. Tsung-yi Lin to Lyman Wynne, August 30, 1966, WHO Archive, M4/87/7 (66), J4.

38. Chen, personal communication.

39. Sartorius, personal communication with author, Geneva, 2010.

40. Bowker and Star, *Sorting Things Out*.

41. Hannah Landecker, "Creeping, Dying, Drinking: The Cinematic Portal and the Microscopic World of the Twentieth-Century Cell," *Science in Context* 24, no. 3 (2011): 381–416.

42. Sander Gilman, Hugh Welch Diamond, John Conolly, and Eric T. Carlson, *The Face of Madness: Hugh W. Diamond and the Origin of Psychiatric Photography*, ed. Sander L. Gilman (New York: Brunner/Mazel, 1976).

43. Quoted in Sander Gilman, *Seeing the Insane* (New York: J. Wiley: Brunner/Mazel, 1982), 166.

44. Georges Didi-Huberman, *Invention of Hysteria: Charcot and the Photographic Iconography of the Salpêtrière* (Cambridge, MA: MIT Press, 2003).

45. Sloan Mahone, "'Hat On—Hat Off': Trauma and Trepanation in Kisii, Western Kenya," *Journal of East African Studies* 8, no. 3 (2014): 331–345.

46. Wellcome Archive, PP/BOW/D4/10 (WHO).

47. Wellcome Archive, PP/BOW/Dr/1 (WHO).

48. "On Making Two Mental Health Films," Wellcome Archive, PP/BOW/5.6/20–22.

49. United Nations Economic and Social Council, "Economics and Social Council: Official Records: Third Year, Seventh Session, Supplement No. 8, Report of the Social Commission," 1948, 28–29.

50. John Bowlby, *Maternal Care and Mental Health* (Geneva: World Health Organization, 1951), 179.

51. Lucien Bovet, *Psychiatric Aspects of Juvenile Delinquency: A Study Prepared on Behalf of the World Health Organization as a Contribution to the United Nations Programme for the Prevention of Crime and Treatment of Offenders* (Geneva: World Health Organization, 1951).

52. Proposed to the World Federation for Mental Health. Thomas L. Pilkington edited the *International Catalogue of World Mental Health Films* in 1962. In correspondence between Pilkington and Peter Baan, August 1966, Pilkington used "World Catalogue of Mental Health Films" to describe his project: WHO Archive, M4/372/8 22.

53. CSA Specialists Meeting on the Adaptation of Education to African Conditions, Lagos, May 23–28, 1960, Contribution to the World Mental Health Year: Recommendations Report.

54. Memorandum on Mental Health Films for the Mental Health Section, World Health Organization, by Dr. Thomas Pilkington, March 18, 1966, WHO Archive, M4/180/12.

55. Man-Horng Lin, "Professor Tsung-yi Lin in Harvard 1950–1952," in *Harvard Alumni Newsletter* (Taipei, 1996), 24–28.

56. E. John Cooper and Norman Sartorius, *A Companion to the Classification of Mental Disorders* (Oxford: Oxford University Press, 2013), 15.

57. Ibid., 12.

58. R. E. Kendell et al., "Diagnostic Criteria of American and British Psychiatrists," *Archives of General Psychiatry* 25, no. 2 (1971).

59. Lyman Wing to Tsung-yi Lin, June 27, 1966, WHO Archive, M4/87/7(66) J4. The "Ditto master" referred to the master copy of a document that could be copied

on a Ditto machine, a duplicating machine common in the twentieth century that was also known as a spirit duplicator.

60. WHO Archive, M4/445/23(65).

61. Alan M. Turing, "Computing Machinery and Intelligence," *Mind* 49 (1950): 433–460.

62. Thomas Rid, *Rise of the Machines: A Cybernetic History* (New York: W. W. Norton, 2016), 54.

63. Christopher Simpson, *Science of Coercion: Communication Research and Psychological Warfare, 1945–1960* (New York: Oxford University Press, 1994); Daniel Pick, *The Pursuit of the Nazi Mind: Hitler, Hess, and the Analysts* (Oxford: Oxford University Press, 2014).

64. Rebecca Lemov, "Brainwashing's Avatar: The Curious Career of Dr. Ewen Cameron," *Grey Room*, no. 45 (2011): 61–87.

65. Warren McCulloch and John Pfeiffer, "On Digital Computers Called Brains," *Science: The Scientific Monthly* 69, no. 6 (1949): 368.

66. Martin Halliwell, "Cold War Ground Zero: Medicine, Psyops and the Bomb," *Journal of American Studies* 44, no. 2 (2010): 313–331.

67. WHO Archive, M4/86/65.

68. Warner V. Slack, "Cybermedicine: How Computing Empowers Doctors and Patients for Better Health Care," *Journal for Healthcare Quality* 25, no. 2 (2003): 52, 53.

69. "Computer in the World of Medicine," *Far East Medical Journal* 3, no. 7 (July 1967): 223.

70. S. H. Lavington, *Early British Computers: The Story of Vintage Computers and the People Who Built Them* (Manchester, UK: Manchester University Press, 1980).

71. IOP/CAM6/7.

72. Capers Jones, *The Technical and Social History of Software Engineering* (Upper Saddle River, NJ: Addison-Wesley, 2014).

73. Paul E. Ceruzzi, *A History of Modern Computing*, 2nd ed. (Cambridge, MA: MIT Press, 2003).

74. J. K. Wing, J. E. Cooper, and N. Sartorius, *Measurement and Classification of Psychiatric Symptoms: An Instruction Manual for the PSE and CATEGO Program* (Cambridge: Cambridge University Press, 1974).

75. Lin, *Road to Psychiatry*, 132.

76. David Baskin, *Computer Applications in Psychiatry and Psychology* (New York: Brunner/Mazel, 1990).

77. Robert L. Spitzer and Joseph L. Fleiss, "A Re-analysis of the Reliability of Psychiatric Diagnosis," *British Journal of Psychiatry* 125 (1974): 341–347.

78. See chapter 11, "Clinical Classification by Computer," IPSS Report, World Health Organization.

79. Lisa Cartwright, *Screening the Body: Tracing Medicine's Visual Culture* (Minneapolis: University of Minnesota Press, 1995).

80. WHO Archive, M4/440/23 (4).

81. Bowker and Star, *Sorting Things Out.*

82. Susan Star and James Griesemer, "Institutional Ecology, 'Translations' and Boundary Objects: Amateurs and Professionals in Berkeley's Museum of Vertebrate Zoology, 1907–39," *Social Studies of Science* 19, no. 3 (1989): 387–420.

83. This was famously described by Star and Griesemer as the important practice of allowing the "trade" of scientific knowledge across boundaries among scientists who speak dissimilar languages. Ibid.

84. Ibid., 393.

85. Lin, *Road to Psychiatry*, 136. For different clustering analysis used in classification of psychiatric diseases, see John S. Strauss, John J. Bartko, and William T. Carpenter, "The Use of Clustering Techniques for the Classification of Psychiatric Patients," *British Journal of Psychiatry* 122, no. 570 (1973): 531–540.

86. Ilana Löwy, "The Strength of Loose Concepts—Boundary Concepts, Federative Experimental Strategies and Disciplinary Growth: The Case of Immunology," *History of Science* 30, no. 4 (December 1, 1992): 371–396.

87. See Assen Jablensky, "Psychiatric Classifications: Validity and Utility," *World Psychiatry* 15, no. 1 (2016): 26–31.

88. Jacques Derrida, *Archive Fever: A Freudian Impression*, trans. Eric Prenowitz (Chicago: University of Chicago Press, 1996).

Chapter 6

1. Assen Jablensky et al., "Schizophrenia: Manifestations, Incidence and Course in Different Cultures: A World Health Organization Ten-Country Study," *Psychological Medicine*, monograph supplement 20 (1992): 1–97; John McGrath, Sukanta Saha, Joy Welham, Ossama El Saadi, Clare MacCauley, and David Chant, "A Systematic Review of the Incidence of Schizophrenia: The Distribution of Rates and the Influence of Sex, Urbanicity, Migrant Status and Methodology," *BMC Medicine* 2, no. 13 (2004), https://doi.org/10.1186/1741-7015-2-13.

2. Martin Roth and H. McClelland, "The Relationship of 'Nuclear' and 'Atypical' Psychoses: Some Proposals for a Classification of Disorders in the Borderlands of

Schizophrenia," *Psychotherapy* 12, no. 1 (1979): 23–54. Also see Kieran McNally, *A Critical History of Schizophrenia* (London: Palgrave Macmillan, 2016).

3. Alex Cohen, Vikram Patel, R. Thara, and Oye Gureje, "Questioning an Axiom: Better Prognosis for Schizophrenia in the Developing World?," *Schizophrenia Bulletin* 34, no. 2 (March 1, 2008): 229–244.

4. Ernest Gruenberg to Tsung-yi Lin, July 7, 1965, WHO Archive, M4/87/7.

5. G. M. Carstairs to Tsung-yi Lin, July 12, 1965, WHO Archive, M4/87/7.

6. WHO Archive WHO/MENT/183, pp. 14, 15.

7. Hans Strotzka to Tsung-yi Lin, February 24, 1966, WHO Archive, M4/440/23 (66).

8. Lorna Wing, "Observations on the Psychiatric Section of the International Classification of Diseases and the British Glossary of Mental Disorders," *Psychological Medicine* 1, no. 1 (1970): 79–95.

9. WHO Archive WHO/MENT/183, p. 17.

10. Eileen M. Brooke, "Do Psychiatric Administrators Need Statisticians?," 1971, Eileen Brooke Papers, AIMG-0799, Box 2.

11. J. K. Wing and Lorna Wing, "Psychotherapy and the National Health Service: An Operational Study," *British Journal of Psychiatry*, no. 116 (1970), 51–55.

12. Vikram Patel, Alex Cohen, R. Thara, and Oye Gureje, "Is the Outcome of Schizophrenia Really Better in Developing Countries?," *Revista Brasileira de Psyquiatria* 28, no. 2 (2006): 149–152.

13. Tsung-yi Lin to Chu-Chang Chen, October 25, 1967, WHO Archive, M4/87/7(67).

14. These terms included autism, hypochondriasis, insight, ambivalence, negativism, change of personality in schizophrenia, schizophrenic thought disorder, and schizophrenic change of affect. John Strauss to Tsung-yi Lin, November 6, 1967, WHO Archive, M4/87/7 (67). For Strauss's legacy, see William Carpenter, "John S. Strauss and Schizophrenia: Early Discovery, Lasting Impact," *American Journal of Psychiatric Rehabilitation* 19, no. 1 (2016): 3–11.

15. For example, "mutism" could be defined operationally as "making no verbal utterances whatsoever," although the word is used in many other ways.

16. Chu-Chang Chen to Tsung-yi Lin, September 27, 1967, WHO Archive, M4 /87/7(67).

17. International Pilot Study of Schizophrenia and World Health Organization, *Schizophrenia: A Multinational Study: A Summary of the Initial Evaluation Phase of the International Pilot Study of Schizophrenia* (Geneva: World Health Organization, 1975).

18. Norman Sartorius, *Understanding the ICD-10 Classification of Mental Disorders: A Pocket Reference* (London: Science Press, 1995).

19. Robert A. Hahn, *Sickness and Healing: An Anthropological Perspective* (New Haven: Yale University Press, 1995).

20. John C. Carothers, *The African Mind in Health and Disease: A Study in Ethnopsychiatry* (Geneva: World Health Organization, 1953). See also chapter 2 of this book.

21. Reuben C. Warren et al., "The Use of Race and Ethnicity in Public Health Surveillance," *Public Health Reports* 109, no. 1 (1994).

22. Arthur Kleinman, "Anthropology and Psychiatry: The Role of Culture in Cross-Cultural Research on Illness," *British Journal of Psychiatry*, no. 151 (1977): 447–454.

23. Ibid.

24. Arthur Kleinman, *Social Origins of Distress and Disease: Depression, Neurasthenia, and Pain in Modern China* (Ann Arbor, MI: UMI Research Press, 1998).

25. Sing Lee, "Diagnosis Postponed: Shenjing Shuairuo and the Transformation of Psychiatry in Post-Mao China," *Culture, Medicine and Psychiatry* 23, no. 3 (1999): 349.

26. By focusing on the symptoms of psychiatric disorders (including schizophrenia and depressive disorders) rather than on the language of diagnoses, the WHO was able to conduct another large epidemiological survey in China with the sponsorship of a French pharmaceutical company in the 1980s. See J. E. Cooper, N. Sartorius, and Yucun Shen, *Mental Disorders in China: Results of the National Epidemiological Survey in 12 Areas* (London: Gaskell, 1996).

27. See Ronald C. Kessler and Bedirhan Ustun, *The WHO World Mental Health Surveys: Global Perspectives on the Epidemiology of Mental Disorders* (New York: Cambridge University Press, 2008).

28. Kenneth L. Pike, *Language in Relation to a Unified Theory of the Structure of Human Behavior* (Berlin: De Gruyter, 1967).

29. James A. Trostle, *Epidemiology and Culture* (New York: Cambridge University Press, 2005).

30. Hsien Rin, "Reflections on the Past Twenty Years," *Bulletin of the Chinese Society of Neurology and Psychiatry* 7, no. 2 (1981): 49–50.

31. Keh-Ming Lin, "Editorial: Psychiatric Research Priorities in Taiwan," *Chinese Psychiatry* 10, no. 3 (1996): 195–196.

32. Emily Baum, *The Invention of Madness: State, Society, and the Insane in Modern China* (Chicago: University of Chicago Press, 2018); Wen-Ji Wang, "An International Teamwork: Mental Hygiene in Shanghai during the 1930s and 1940s," *History of Psychology* 22, no. 4 (2019): 289–309; Peter Szto, "Psychiatric Space and Design

Antecedents: The John G. Kerr Refuge for the Insane," in *Psychiatry and Chinese History*, ed. Howard Chiang (London: Pickering & Chatto, 2014), 71–90.

33. C. Y. Wu, "Psychiatry in the People's Republic of China," *World Mental Health* 12, no. 2 (May 1960): 73–75.

34. Tsung-yi Lin and Leon Eisenberg, eds., *Mental Health Planning for One Billion People: A Chinese Perspective* (Vancouver: University of British Columbia Press, 1985).

35. Ibid.

36. The first *CCMD* appeared in 1979. A revised classification, the *CCMD-1*, was made available in 1981 and further modified in 1984 (*CCMD-2-R*). The *CCMD-3* was published in 2001. See Sing Lee, "From Diversity to Unity: The Classification of Mental Disorders in 21st-Century China," *Psychiatric Clinics of North America* 24, no. 3 (2001): 421–431.

37. Ibid.

38. In 1982, the World Health Organization established another collaborating center with Shanghai Mental Health Center to focus on the training of psychiatric specialists. The center was formerly Puci Rehabilitation Hospital, founded in 1935 in Shanghai.

39. As compared to the *DSM* system, the ICD is favored in China as it has been developed for underdeveloped countries. See Yan-Fang Chen, "Chinese Classification of Mental Disorders (Ccmd-3): Towards Integration in International Classification," *Psychopathology*, no. 35 (2002): 171–175; Sing Lee, "Cultures in Psychiatric Nosology: The CCMD-2-R and International Classification of Mental Disorders," *Culture, Medicine and Psychiatry* 20, no. 4 (1996): 421–472.

40. Sing Lee, "Higher Earnings, Bursting Trains and Exhausted Bodies: The Creation of Travelling Psychosis in Post-Reform China," *Social Science & Medicine* 47, no. 9 (1998): 1247–1261.

41. See Nancy N. Chen, *Breathing Spaces: Qigong, Psychiatry, and Healing in China* (New York: Columbia University Press, 2003); David A. Palmer, *Qigong Fever: Body, Science, and Utopia in China* (New York: Columbia University Press, 2007).

42. Human Rights Watch, *Dangerous Minds: Political Psychiatry in China Today and Its Origins in the Mao Era* (Hilversum, Netherlands: Human Rights Watch; Geneva Initiative on Psychiatry, 2002).

43. Yucun Shen, "The Significance of Developing Psychiatric Epidemiological Studies," *Chinese Journal of Psychiatry* 31, no. 2 (1998): 67–68.

44. Weixin Zhang, Yucun Shen, and Shuran Li, "Psychiatric Epidemiological Studies in Seven Regions in China," *Chinese Journal of Psychiatry* 31, no. 2 (1998): 69–71.

45. Arthur Kleinman, "Neurasthenia and Depression: A Study of Somatization and Culture in China," *Culture, Medicine, and Psychiatry* 6, no. 2 (1982): 117–190.

46. Sing Lee, "Depression: Coming of Age in China," in *Deep China: The Moral Life of the Person*, ed. Arthur Kleinman (Berkeley: University of California Press, 2011), 177–212. Also see Sing Lee and Arthur Kleinman, "Are Somatoform Disorders Changing with Time? The Case of Neurasthenia in China," *Psychosomatic Medicine* 69, no. 9 (2007): 846–849.

47. Byron Good and Mary-Jo Delvecchio Good, "Significance of the 686 Program for China and for Global Mental Health," *Shanghai Archives of Psychiatry* 24, no. 3 (2012): 175–177.

48. Yueqin Huang et al., "The China Mental Health Survey (CMHS): I. Background, Aims and Measures," *Social Psychiatry and Psychiatric Epidemiology* 51, no. 11 (November 2016): 1559–1569.

49. Kam-Shing Yip, *Mental Health Service in the People's Republic of China* (New York: Nova Science Publisher, 2007).

50. Dorothy Porter and UC Medical Humanities Consortium, *Health Citizenship: Essays in Social Medicine and Biomedical Politics* (Berkeley: University of California Medical Humanities Press, 2011).

51. Shiyu Wang and Xuyang Xuan, "Zhengzhou Orders to Identify Two Mentally Ill Individuals out of 1000," *Sina News*, last modified October 9, 2013, http://news.sina.com.cn/c/2013-10-09/094128383609.shtml.

52. Sunil S. Amrith, *Decolonizing International Health: India and Southeast Asia, 1930–65* (Basingstoke, UK: Palgrave Macmillan, 2006).

53. Javed Siddiqi, *World Health and World Politics: The World Health Organization and the UN System* (Columbia: University of South Carolina Press, 1995), 147–192.

54. John Farley, "The Interim Commission, 1946–48: The Long Wait," in *Brock Chisholm, the World Health Organization, and the Cold War* (Vancouver: University of British Columbia Press, 2008), 186.

55. For example, see Randall M. Packard, "Postcolonial Medicine," in *Medicine in the Twentieth Century*, ed. Roger Cooter and John V. Pickstone (Amsterdam: Harwood Academic, 2000).

56. Farley, "The Interim Commission, 1946–48," 186–187.

57. Hui-Ling Hu, "Passport," in *Daoyu Ailian (Love Stories on the Island)*, ed. Hui-Ling Hu (Taipei: Yu-Shan Books, 1995).

58. Marnie Copland, *A Lin Odyssey* (New Orleans: Paraclete Press, 1987), 136. After he left the WHO in 1969, Lin first lived in Michigan in the United States

and eventually settled in Vancouver, Canada, where he lived until his death in 2010.

59. Charles E. Allen, "World Health and World Politics," *International Organizations*, no. 4 (1950): 27–43.

60. Micahel Borrus, Dieter Ernst, and Stephen Haggard, eds., *International Production Networks in Asia: Rivalry or Riches* (New York: Routledge, 2001).

61. See Randall M. Packard, "The Making of a Tropical Disease: A Short History of Malaria," *Emerging Infectious Diseases* 14, no. 10 (2008): 1679–1679.

62. Ibid. See also Siddiqi, *World Health and World Politics.*

63. See Centers for Disease Control and Prevention, "Malaria Eradication in Taiwan," in *The Executive Yuan Department of Health* (Taipei: Centers for Disease Control Prevention, Dept. of Health, The Executive Yuan, Republic of China [Taiwan], 2005), xxii, 300.

64. See Pow-Meng Yap, "Words and Things in Comparative Psychiatry, with Special Reference to the Exotic Psychoses," *Acta Psychiatrica Scandinavica*, no. 38 (1962): 157–182.

65. Narendra Wig, "Problems of Mental Health in India," *Journal of Clinical Social Psychiatry*, no. 17 (1960).

66. Keum Young Chun Pang, "Hwabyung: The Construction of a Korean Popular Illness among Korean Elderly Immigrant Women in the United States," *Culture, Medicine and Psychiatry*, no. 14 (1990): 495–512.

67. Pow-Meng Yap, "Koro—A Culture-Bound Depersonalization Syndrome," *British Journal of Psychiatry*, no. 111 (1965): 43–50; Ivan Crozier, "Making up Koro: Multiplicity, Psychiatry, Culture, and Penis-Shrinking Anxieties," *Journal of the History of Medicine and Allied Sciences* 67, no. 1 (2011): 36–70; Howard Chiang, "Translating Culture and Psychiatry across the Pacific: How Koro Became Culture-bound," *History of Science* 53 (2015): 102–119.

68. Robert L. Winzeler, *Latah in Southeast Asia: The History and Ethnography of a Culture-Bound Syndrome* (Cambridge: Cambridge University Press), 1995.

69. For *hsieh-ping*, *frigophobia*, and *utox*, see Tsung-yi Lin, "A Study of the Incidence of Mental Disorder in Chinese and Other Cultures," *Psychiatry*, no. 15 (1953): 313–336; Y. H. Chang, H. Rin, and C. C. Chen, "Frigophobia: A Report of Five Cases," *Bulletin of the Chinese Society of Neurology and Psychiatry* 1, no. 2 (1975): 13. For Tseng's handbook, see Wen-Shing Tseng, *Handbook of Cultural Psychiatry* (San Diego: Academic Press, 2001).

70. Hsien Rin, *The Gift of Cultural Psychiatry: From Japan to Taiwan* (Taipei: PsyGarden, 2007); Wen-Shing Tseng, *One Life, Three Cultures: The Self-Analysis on Personality Shaped by China, Japan and America* (Taipei: Psychology Press, 2010).

71. Hahn, *Sickness and Healing.*

72. Kleinman, "Anthropology and Psychiatry."

73. Emmanuel Delille, "Eric Wittkower and the Foundation of Montreal's Transcultural Psychiatry Research Unit after World War II," *History of Psychiatry* 29, no. 3 (2018): 282–296, https://doi.org/10.1177/0957154X18765417.

74. See Laurence J. Kirmayer, "50 Years of Transcultural Psychiatry," *Transcultural Psychiatry* 50, no. 1 (April 2013): 3–5.

75. Allan V. Horwitz and Jerome C. Wakefield, *The Loss of Sadness: How Psychiatry Transformed Normal Sorrow into Depressive Disorder* (New York: Oxford University Press, 2012).

76. Hahn, *Sickness and Healing,* 13–39.

77. Ibid., 32.

78. Renato D. Alarcón, "Culture, Cultural Factors and Psychiatric Diagnosis: Review and Projections," *World Psychiatry* 8, no. 3 (October 2009): 131–139, http://www.ncbi.nlm.nih.gov/pmc/articles/PMC2755270/.

79. Julian Leff, personal communication with the author, London, 2010.

80. Chu-Chang Chen, personal communication with the author, Taipei, 2011.

81. Donna C. Mehos and Suzanne Moon, "The Uses of Portability: Circulating Experts in the Technopolitics of Cold War and Decolonization," in *Entangled Geographies: Empire and Technopolitics in the Global Cold War,* ed. Gabrielle Hecht (Cambridge, MA: MIT Press, 2011).

82. See ibid.

83. See John Farley, *Brock Chisholm, the World Health Organization, and the Cold War* (Vancouver: University of British Columbia Press, 2008).

84. Tsung-yi Lin, *Road to Psychiatry: Across the East and the West* (Taipei: Daw Shiang Publishing, 1994).

85. Wei-tsun Soong, personal communication with author (Chiayi City, 2011).

86. Robert Van Voren, *Cold War in Psychiatry: Human Factors, Secret Actors* (Leiden: Brill, 2010).

87. The first case of Taiwan sending delegates to prevent the Communists' participation in international medical conferences was in December 1956, after the Ministry of Foreign Affairs was informed that a delegate of "pseudo China" was liaising with the organizers of a conference on ophthalmology. See National Security to Ministry of Foreign Affairs, December 28, 1956, Academia Historica, index no. 172-4, vol. 0044-2, 020000021163A.

88. For example, in recent years, working groups and conferences have been organized to study the history and anthropology of international psychiatric epidemiology and global mental health. Some of their works have already been published, such as the special issue "History of Psychiatric Epidemiology," *International Journal of Epidemiology* 43, suppl. 1 (August 2014), https://academic.oup.com/ije/issue/43/suppl_1.

89. Anne M. Lovell, "The World Health Organization and the Contested Beginnings of Psychiatry Epidemiology as an International Discipline: One Rope, Many Strands," *International Journal of Epidemiology* 43, suppl. 1 (2014): 16–18.

90. WHO Archive, WFMH/IC, 6/7 P.12(111).

91. Norman Sartorius to Co. Ian A. A. Quenum, Regional Director, AFRO, September 6, 1976, WHO Archive, M4/86/38.

92. Shunsuke Tsurumi, *An Intellectual History of Wartime Japan, 1931–1945* (London: KPI, 1986).

Epilogue

1. See China Mills, "Global Psychiatrization and Psychic Colonization: The Coloniality of Global Mental Health," in *Critical Inquiries for Social Justice in Mental Health*, ed. Marina Morrow and Lorraine Halinka Malcoe (Toronto: University of Toronto Press, 2017), 87–109.

2. Anne Harrington, *Mind Fixers: Psychiatry's Troubled Search for the Biology of Mental Illness* (New York: W. W. Norton, 2019).

3. Stefan Ecks, "Commentary: Ethnographic Critiques of Global Mental Health," *Transcultural Psychiatry* 53, no. 6 (2016): 804–808.

4. M. Prince et al., "No Health without Mental Health," *The Lancet* 370, no. 9590 (September 8, 2007): 859–877.

5. Howard Higginbotham, *Third World Challenge to Psychiatry: Culture Accommodation and Mental Health Care* (Honolulu: East-West Center by the University of Hawaii Press, 1984).

6. Ecks, "Commentary."

7. D. Satcher, "Global Mental Health: Its Time Has Come," *JAMA* 285, no. 13 (2001): 1697.

8. Vikram Patel, "Why Mental Health Matters to Global Health," *Transcultural Psychiatry* 51, no. 6 (2014): 777–789.

9. Anthony Pagden, *Peoples and Empires* (London: Weidenfeld & Nicolson, 2001).

10. Nitsan Chorev, *The World Health Organization between North and South* (Ithaca, NY: Cornell University Press, 2012).

11. Nayan Chanda, *Bound Together: How Traders, Preachers, Adventurers, and Warriors Shaped Globalization* (New Haven: Yale University Press, 2007).

12. R. Giel and T. W. Harding, "Psychiatric Priorities in Developing Countries," *British Journal of Psychiatry* 128 (June 1976): 513–522.

13. Higginbotham, *Third World Challenge to Psychiatry.*

14. Yolana Pringle, *Psychiatry and Decolonization in Uganda* (London: Palgrave Macmillan, 2018).

15. WHO Expert Committee on Mental Health and World Health Organization, *Organization of Mental Health Services in Developing Countries: Sixteenth Report of the WHO Expert Committee on Mental Health* (meeting held in Geneva, October 22–28, 1974) (Geneva: World Health Organization, 1975).

16. Anne M. Lovell, Ursula M. Read, and Claudia Lang, "Genealogies and Anthropologies of Global Mental Health," *Culture, Medicine, and Psychiatry* 43, no. 4 (2019): 519–547.

17. Didier Fassin, "That Obscure Object of Global Health," in *Medical Anthropology at the Intersections: History, Activisms, and Futures,* ed. Marcia C. Inhorn and Emily A. Wentzell (Durham: Duke University Press, 2012), 95–115.

18. Erich Fromm, *The Sane Society* (New York: Holt, Rinehart and Winston, 1995), 72.

19. Theodore M. Brown, "The World Health Organization and the Transition from 'International' to 'Global' Public Health," *American Journal of Public Health* 96, no. 1 (January 2006): 62–72.

20. See Tanya Luhrman, introduction to *Our Most Troubling Madness: Case Studies in Schizophrenia across Cultures,* ed. Tanya Luhrman and Jocelyn Marrow (Oakland: University of California Press, 2016), 1–26; Holla Bharath and Jagadisha Thirthalli, "Course and Outcome of Schizophrenia in Asian Countries: Review of Research in the Past Three Decades," *Asian Journal of Psychiatry* 14 (2015): 3–12; and P. Kulhara, R. Shah, and S. Grover, "Is the Course and Outcome of Schizophrenia Better in the 'Developing' World?," *Asian Journal of Psychiatry* 2 (2009): 55–62.

21. J. W. Keeley et al., "Developing a Science of Clinical Utility in Diagnostic Classification Systems Field Study Strategies for ICD-11 Mental and Behavioral Disorders," *American Psychologist* 71, no. 1 (January 2016): 3–16, doi: 10.1037/a0039972.

22. Geoffrey Pleyers, *Alter-Globalization: Becoming Actors in a Global Age* (New York: Wiley, 2011).

23. Griet Cuypere and Sam Winter, "A Gender Incongruence Diagnosis: Where to Go?," *The Lancet* 3, no. 9 (September 1, 2016): 796–797, https://www.thelancet.com/journals/lanpsy/article/PIIS2215-0366(16)30212-7/abstract.

24. Geoffrey M. Reed et al., "Disorders Related to Sexuality and Gender Identity in the ICD-11: Revising the ICD-10 Classification Based on Current Scientific Evidence, Best Clinical Practices, and Human Rights Considerations," *World Psychiatry* 15, no. 3 (October 2016): 205–221, https://www.ncbi.nlm.nih.gov/pmc/articles/PMC5032510/.

25. World Health Organization, *International Statistical Classification of Diseases and Related Health Problems*, 11th ed. (2018), https://www.who.int/classifications/icd/en/, retrieved from https://icd.who.int/browse11/l-m/en.

26. See Yichen Rao, "From Confucianism to Psychology: Rebooting the Internet Addicts in China," *History of Psychology* 22 (2019).

27. Robert Aronowitz, *Making Sense of Illness: Science, Society, and Disease* (Cambridge: Cambridge University Press, 1998).

28. Michael Ward, *Quantifying the World: UN Ideas and Statistics* (Bloomington: Indiana University Press, 2004.)

29. Norman Sartorius, A. Jablensky, and D. A. Reigier, *Sources and Traditions of Classification in Psychiatry* (Bern: Hogrefe and Huber, 1990), 2.

30. World Health Organization, *International Classification of Diseases for Mortality and Morbidity Statistics*, 11th ed. (Geneva: World Health Organization, 2018).

31. See Kenneth Kendler, "Alternative Futures for the DSM Revision Process: Iteration V. Paradigm Shift," *British Journal of Psychiatry* 197 (2010): 263–265.

32. See Aihwa Ong, "(Re)Articulations of Citizenship," *Political Science and Politics* 38, no. 4 (2005): 697–699.

Index